THIS IS

REALLY

WAR

To Eleanor

THE INCREDIBLE TRUE STORY

THIS IS

OF A NAVY NURSE POW

REALLY

IN THE OCCUPIED PHILIPPINES

WAR

EMILIE LE BEAU LUCCHESI

Reveal the 12 amhr!

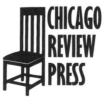
CHICAGO
REVIEW
PRESS

Emilie Lucchesi

Published by Chicago Review Press Incorporated
814 North Franklin Street
Chicago, Illinois 60610
ISBN 978-1-64160-076-7

Library of Congress Cataloging-in-Publication Data
Names: Lucchesi, Emilie Le Beau, author.
Title: This is really war : the incredible true story of a Navy nurse POW in
    the occupied Philippines / Emilie Le Beau Lucchesi.
Description: Chicago, Illinois : Chicago Review Press, [2019] | Includes
    bibliographical references and index.
Identifiers: LCCN 2018058584 (print) | LCCN 2019002844 (ebook) | ISBN
    9781641600774 (PDF edition) | ISBN 9781641600798 (EPUB edition) | ISBN
    9781641600781 (Kindle edition) | ISBN 9781641600767 (cloth edition)
Subjects: LCSH: Danner, Dorothy Still, 1914–2001. | Women prisoners
    of war—Philippines—Biography. | United States. Navy—Nurses—
    Biography. | United States. Navy—Officers—Biography. | Los Baños
    Internment Camp. | World War, 1939–1945—Prisoners and prisons,
    Japanese. | World War, 1939–1945—Philippines. | Philippines—
    History—Japanese occupation, 1942–1945.
Classification: LCC D805.P6 (ebook) | LCC D805.P6 L83 2019 (print) |
    DDC 940.54/7092 [B] —dc23
LC record available at https://lccn.loc.gov/2018058584

Typesetting: Nord Compo
Map design: Chris Erichsen

Printed in the United States of America
5 4 3 2 1

For my grandfather Leon J. Le Beau, PhD. US Army,
5th Medical Laboratory, South Pacific

And always, my husband, Michael Lucchesi, for many, many reasons

Contents

_____

Author's Note

N O DIALOGUE WAS re-created for this book. Quotations were sourced from oral histories, interview transcripts, memoirs, and other documented sources.

Key Figures

The "Twelve Anchors"

The dozen nurses who served in the Santo Tomas and Los Baños prisoner of war camps as of January 1942. All but Basilia Torres Steward were members of the Navy Nurse Corps.

DOROTHY STILL: California native who was twenty-seven years old and near the end of her two-year assignment in the Philippines when Cavite was bombed. Had orders to return to the United States on January 1, 1942.

MARY FRANCES CHAPMAN: Twenty-eight years old, recently engaged; had submitted her resignation to the navy. Planned to return to her family in Chicago while waiting for her fiancé to finish his service.

LAURA M. COBB: Chief nurse. Longtime veteran of the navy who was strict with her nurses but fiercely protected them when she was able to do so. Almost fifty years old; originally from Kansas.

BERTHA EVANS: Thirty-seven years old. Also trained as a dietitian. Originally from Oregon; recently engaged.

HELEN C. GORZELANSKI: Thirty-four years old; from Nebraska.

MARY ROSE HARRINGTON: Considered "an Irish beauty," with auburn
    hair. Native of South Dakota. Moved her widowed mother to San
    Diego after she enlisted. Age twenty-eight.

MARGARET "PEG" NASH: Thirty years old; recently engaged. Originally
    from Wilkes-Barre, Pennsylvania. Petite, energetic, and bright.

GOLDIA O'HAVER: Age thirty-nine; from Iowa. Practical and efficient
    yet warm in personality. Also trained as a surgical nurse.

ELDENE PAIGE: Turned twenty-eight on the day of the Cavite bombing.
    Originally from South Dakota but raised in Southern California.
    Petite, shy, and kind.

SUSIE PITCHER: Born in Iowa in 1901. Nurse anesthetist who had been
    in the navy for more than a decade. Heavy smoker; living with
    emphysema.

BASILIA TORRES STEWARD: Twenty-eight years old. Filipina married
    to an American naval officer. Served alongside the navy nurses
    throughout their captivity.

CARRIE EDWINA TODD: California native who had the same assign-
    ment as Dorothy Still and was expecting new orders. Known as
    Edwina; age thirty at time of capture.

Other Medical Personnel

ANN BERNATITUS: Navy nurse with surgical experience. Became the
    only nurse from Cavite to escape imprisonment after the army
    requested her service and then evacuated her to Australia.

DANA NANCE, MD: Civilian. Surgeon at Los Baños prison camp.

GWENDOLYN L. HENSHAW: Army nurse POW; native of California.
    Reunited with fellow nursing school graduate Dorothy Still at
    Santo Tomas prison camp.

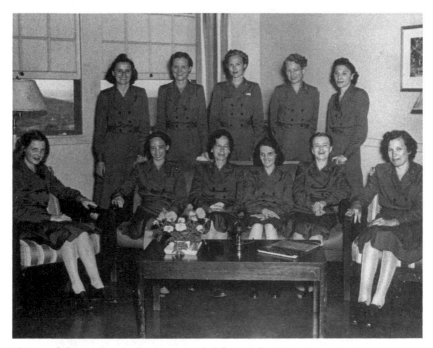

Eleven of the twelve anchors. *Seated, left to right:* Mary Rose Harrington, Eldene Paige, Laura Cobb, Peg Nash, Edwina Todd, Bertha Evans. *Standing, left to right:* Mary Chapman, Goldia O'Haver, Dorothy Still, Susie Pitcher, Helen Gorzelanski. *Not pictured:* Basilia Torres Steward. *Courtesy of Bureau of Medicine and Surgery*

Chronology

___

1937

NOVEMBER: Dorothy Still applies to the Navy Nurse Corps after seeing an article in the *American Journal of Nursing*.

DECEMBER: Dorothy joins the navy and is assigned to San Diego.

1940

JANUARY: Dorothy transfers to Cavite Naval Base at Cañacao, Philippines.

1941

SUMMER: US Navy orders all spouses and dependents to return to the United States.

DECEMBER 7: Pearl Harbor is attacked by the Japanese.

DECEMBER 8: US Congress declares war on Japan.

DECEMBER 10: Japan attacks Cavite Naval Base in Philippines.

DECEMBER 11: Dorothy and the other navy nurses are evacuated to
Manila.

DECEMBER 26: General MacArthur declares Manila an "open city." US
and Filipino forces evacuate Manila for Bataan and Corregidor.

1942

JANUARY 2: Dorothy and ten other navy nurses are taken prisoners of
war. Chief Nurse Laura Cobb allows civilian nurse Basilia Torres
Steward to be absorbed into the group.

MARCH 8: Dorothy and the other navy nurse POWs are transferred to
Santo Tomas, a former college converted into a prison camp.

APRIL 9: Bataan falls.

MAY 3: Navy nurse Ann Bernatitus escapes on an army submarine.

MAY 6: Corregidor falls.

JULY 2: Army nurses are brought to Santo Tomas prison camp but segregated from the general population. Dorothy reunites with her
school friend Gwendolyn Henshaw.

AUGUST 25: Army nurses are integrated with rest of the population.

1943

MAY 14: The eleven navy nurses transfer to Los Baños prison camp
with 788 male inmates.

1944

OCTOBER 20: General MacArthur lands on the Philippine island of
Leyte and announces, "I have returned."

DECEMBER 14: Prisoners are massacred at Palawan prisoner of war
camp.

1945

FEBRUARY 3: Santo Tomas is liberated.

FEBRUARY 23: Los Baños is liberated.

MARCH 10: Dorothy and the other navy nurses arrive in mainland
United States.

JULY 5: Philippines is completely liberated.

AUGUST 15: Japan surrenders.

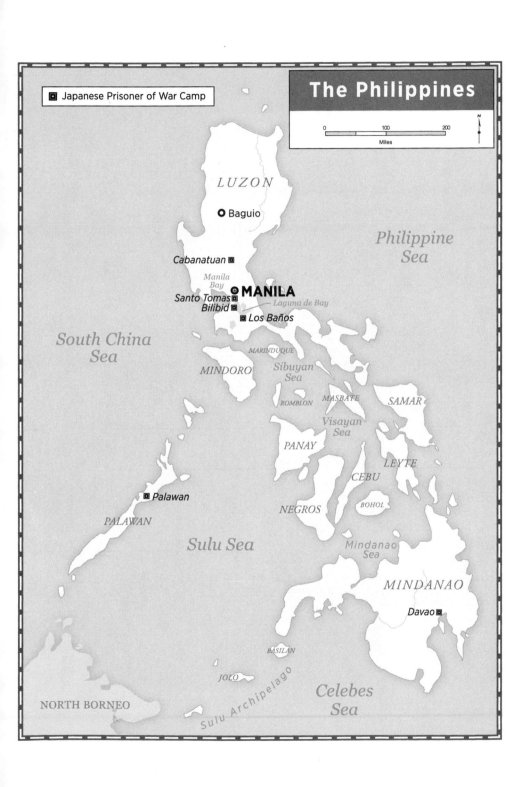

The Philippines

Japanese Prisoner of War Camp

0 — 100 — 200
Miles

N

LUZON

○ Baguio

Cabanatuan ▣

Manila Bay

○**MANILA**

Santo Tomas ▣
Bilibid ▣
▣ Los Baños

Laguna de Bay

Philippine Sea

South China Sea

MARINDUQUE

MINDORO

Sibuyan Sea

ROMBLON

MASBATE

SAMAR

Visayan Sea

PANAY

LEYTE

CEBU

NEGROS

BOHOL

▣ Palawan

PALAWAN

Sulu Sea

Mindanao Sea

MINDANAO

Davao ▣

BASILAN

JOLO

Sulu Archipelago

NORTH BORNEO

Celebes Sea

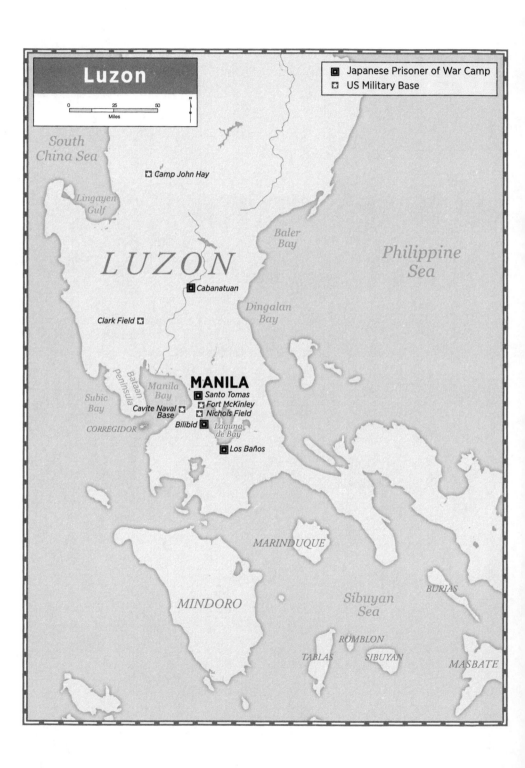

Luzon

Miles
0 — 25 — 50

N

Japanese Prisoner of War Camp
US Military Base

South China Sea

★ Camp John Hay

Lingayen Gulf

LUZON

Baler Bay

Philippine Sea

■ Cabanatuan

Dingalan Bay

Clark Field ★

Bataan Peninsula

Manila Bay

Subic Bay

MANILA
■ Santo Tomas
★ Fort McKinley
★ Nichols Field

Cavite Naval Base ★

CORREGIDOR

Bilibid ■

Laguna de Bay

■ Los Baños

MARINDUQUE

MINDORO

Sibuyan Sea

BURIAS

ROMBLON

TABLAS   *SIBUYAN*

MASBATE

Part I

1941

———

1

I'd Die Before
I Wore Those

DOROTHY STILL SLEPT soundly in her bed in the nurses' quarters. It was comfortably dark, and a breeze flowed through the veranda attached to her private room. She did not stir as the telephone rang downstairs, sending a shrill scream through the quiet house. Dietitian Bertha Evans picked up the handset and heard her fiancé's voice on the other end of the extension. He was an officer assigned to the nearby naval yard in Cañacao, Philippines, and he was calling with urgent news.

"Bertha," he said. "Pearl Harbor has been bombed. We've been up all night with the admiral."

The US armed forces in the Philippines anticipated they would be next. At one point during the night, radar had detected a formation near Manila Bay. Warhawks took to the sky to intercept the threat, but no contact had been made.

Bertha knew she had to wake her superior, Chief Nurse Laura M. Cobb. She hurried up the stairs and knocked on Cobb's door. "We're at war with Japan," she reported.

Doorways began to crack as the other women heard the commotion. Cobb instinctively knew a blackout order was in effect. "Do not turn on your lights," she warned.

Nurse Mary Rose Harrington squinted in the darkness. Cobb ordered her to dress and accompany her to receive orders. Dorothy continued to sleep through the disturbances. She didn't hear Cobb and Mary Rose return to the quarters. Nor did she wake when Mary Rose clanked around the kitchen, looking to start a pot of coffee. Dorothy finally opened her eyes when the auburn-haired woman stood over her bed.

"Dottie! Wake up!" Mary Rose urged.

Dorothy stumbled from bed and followed Mary Rose. The other nurses stood in the darkened hallway, stunned and confused. Cobb was brief. All they knew for certain was Japan had attacked Pearl Harbor around midnight Manila time. It would be only a matter of hours before Congress officially declared war. But what did that mean to the nurses? Should they expect an attack as well? Cobb didn't know. She ordered her nurses into uniform.

Dorothy felt her way back to her room. She went to her washbasin and turned on the water, thinking about newspaper reports describing the fighting in Europe. She had seen photos of decimated villages and images of destroyed battlefields. Would war in the South Pacific look the same? Dorothy thought not. If there was indeed a war with Japan, she assumed the United States would quickly win. It wasn't the same as the hostilities between the Europeans.

Dorothy opened her dresser drawers and selected a pair of white knee-high tights. She stepped into the white dress, fixing the buttons that ran down to the high-waist belt. She combed back her blond hair and secured her striped cap to her head. Dorothy pulled her flashlight from the box and screwed off the bottom. She slipped in two batteries and then felt the spring press tighten as she rotated the end back into place. After masking the top with blue cellophane so it was safe to use

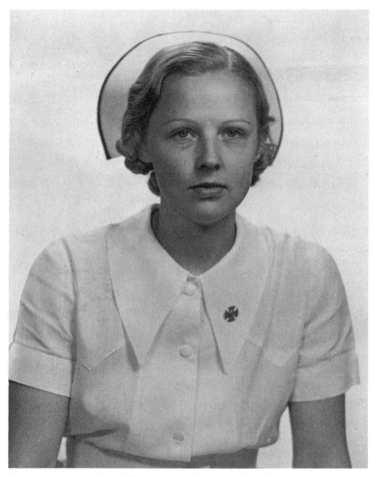

Navy nurse Dorothy Still. *Courtesy of Bureau of Medicine and Surgery*

in a blackout, she shone the light on her mirror and felt unnerved as she studied her reflection in the ghostly blue light.

Dorothy joined the other nurses in the living room. The women traded mixed expressions of doubt and reassurance. Several of the nurses didn't think the Asiatic Fleet was prepared for battle. Others thought the same as Dorothy—Japan was a small nation and it was no match for the mighty United States. Susie Pitcher, a forty-year-old nurse anesthetist from Des Moines, lit a cigarette. Susie loved smoking and seemed determined to not let her emphysema interfere with her favorite pastime.

Susie inhaled and released a swirling cloud as she spoke. "You girls ready for war?" she asked.

The young nurses weren't sure what to think. Earlier in 1941, the navy had begun censoring mail, and spouses and dependents of military personnel had been shipped back to the States. At the time, the nurses felt odd to be the only women on base, but then they adjusted to the new routine. Blackouts and air raid drills became standard, yet with all the warnings and preparation, nothing ever happened. Now it was difficult to determine whether they should truly be alarmed.

It was easy, however, to feel vulnerable. The naval base was located on a small peninsula just south of Manila. The peninsula had an odd shape, like a crab's claw. The navy occupied the parts that resembled the pinchers, filling the area around the bay with an ammunition depot, hospital, living quarters, and a naval yard to service marine vessels. There were also two soaring radio towers, which the nurses detested for being an easy target. What would happen if they were bombed? The women shuddered to think, especially if the ammunitions depot took a direct hit. The concussion could obliterate the entire peninsula.

Several of the nurses didn't want to face the possibility of war. But others, like Bertha, experienced ominous warnings and sensed the time had come. Bertha had transferred to the Philippines in February. On the boat ride to Hawaii, a reserve officer said he felt sorry for her.

"You'll be eating fish heads and rice before you come home," he warned.

"Do you really think so?" Bertha asked.

"I know so," he cautioned.

The comment stuck with Bertha. At thirty-seven years old, she had been in the navy for a decade. She had wavy brown hair and beautiful dark eyes that turned downward at the corners. Most sailors typically boasted in an attempt to impress her. The reserve officer's lack of bravado felt like a chilling omen.

The women came to attention as Cobb entered the room. She reported they did not have specific orders from the admiral. However, the fleet surgeon had told Cobb they needed to evacuate the hospital. The women were to report immediately for duty. Dorothy followed the other nurses into the humid air. Rain had fallen overnight and the ground was spotted with puddles. Cobb instructed the nurses to run to the hospital as if they were under attack.

Dorothy and the other women began to jog without much enthusiasm. In the distance, a pathologist stood outside the hospital and watched the pack of approaching blue lights. He wondered how long it would take the nurses to run the two-block distance. If the base was hit, how quickly could the nurses arrive? He pulled out a stopwatch and began to time them.

The nurses were hesitant in the dark. As they approached, the pathologist saw they were trying to avoid splashing in the puddles. The nurses did not want to get their shoes wet or their uniforms dirty. They took the long way around larger pools of water and carefully stepped over smaller puddles, sometimes stopping to hold on to each other for support. The pathologist looked at the second hand spinning around the dial. What were these nurses doing? Had they no sense of urgency?

The pathologist held up the stopwatch as Dorothy and the other nurses trotted up the circular drive. "Two minutes and twenty-three seconds," he scolded.

War was not what Arissa Still had intended for her daughter when she brought Dorothy to the Los Angeles County General Hospital for an interview with the nursing school. It was 1932, and Arissa knew people who had lost their jobs and then their homes. She wanted her daughter to find a stable career, and Dorothy had failed to supply one practical idea of which her mother approved. Dorothy had dreamily proposed working as a costume designer in Hollywood. The girl could sew, yes, and she appreciated fashion, but Arissa thought Hollywood was unpredictable and competitive.

Nursing, Arissa had assumed, was a far safer choice. The Los Angeles County General Hospital offered a three-year program with free tuition, room, and board. The student nurses worked at the hospital and received a small monthly stipend. Being paid to go to school? At a time when unemployment was near 25 percent? Arissa promptly brought Dorothy in for an interview and hovered in the hallway while her daughter met with the admissions director. She knew her daughter was an excellent candidate. Dorothy had performed well at Burbank High School, and she was one of a few students with enough merit points to join an exclusive honorary. The nursing school officials were impressed, as Arissa expected.

Arissa's plan for her daughter was on track—until Dorothy graduated and received her pin. Then Arissa realized nurses were not immune from the crippled economy. Low wages and job insecurity were standard, and nurses typically bounced from one short contract to the next. In the first two years after graduation, Dorothy cycled through three jobs. The last of these was at a small hospital in a desert town where a few senior nurses successfully campaigned to have Dorothy and another young nurse fired. Demoralized, Dorothy returned to her parents' home and looked for a new position.

Dorothy flipped through the November 1937 issue of the *American Journal of Nursing* and stopped on an article about the Federal Nursing Services. Its military nurses enjoyed the "security of a regular salary," the article promised. They also received medical care, four weeks' leave, and the opportunity to train in a specialty. Dorothy was intrigued, but she still stung from her recent termination. She figured she was wasting a stamp when she wrote to request an application. Within a month, she received notification that the navy was indeed interested. Before the year was over, Dorothy was instructed to report to duty in San Diego as a member of the Navy Nurse Corps.

As Dorothy reported to San Diego, the world was becoming increasingly unstable. The United States maintained an isolationist stance, but American military commanders watched with unease as Japan conquered Nanking, the capital city of China, on December 13, 1937. Within mere weeks, more than 250,000 Chinese were massacred by the Japanese army. It seemed that every newspaper in the United States had a front-page story about the invasion, but few Americans understood the extent of the massacre. Chinese men, women, and children were rounded up, marched through the streets, and then sadistically executed. Every type of agony emerged in Nanking. Yet American attention instead focused on the sinking of a naval ship on a river near Nanking. President Franklin D. Roosevelt demanded an apology and payment, both of which Japan supplied. The US government then edited the news footage. When newsreels spun in cinemas across the county, Americans were treated to a sanitized account of the violence, as well as a false sense that Japan knew better than to mess with Uncle Sam.

The world was darkening, and the United States simply wasn't ready to defend itself. In 1937, the annual report of the secretary of war to the president described the country's forces as a "peace time army." Just one year later, the authors of the report were looking long and hard at their own inadequacies. With only about 162,000 enlisted men, the US military was merely the eighteenth largest in the world. The report also admitted that after the recent World War, the United States failed to keep pace with the development of defensive weapons. Materials shortages during the Great Depression added more budgetary challenges, and the military was woefully short on antiaircraft defenses. As for aircraft, the report authors pitifully described themselves as making "progress."

At the end of 1939, Dorothy learned that she was being transferred from San Diego to the Philippines. She was to report before February 1, 1940, to Cavite Naval Base. Dorothy promptly consulted a map and anxiously scanned the distance across the Pacific Ocean and into the Philippine Sea. She had never left the United States, and the Philippines seemed so far away. The other nurses helped to ease her anxiety. They recommended that Dorothy pack plenty of party dresses. Nurses at Cavite were only required to work half shifts due to the high temperatures, so Dorothy would have plenty of time to play tennis, golf, swim, and enjoy evenings out with officers. She was assured it was a very good assignment.

Dorothy eased her own anxiety by visiting the library in her Southern California hometown of Long Beach during her two-week leave. She read about the history of the Philippines and its quest for independence, which gave her an admiration for the Filipino people. The Spanish had colonized the archipelago in the sixteenth century. After the Spanish-American War in the late 1890s, the United States took over foreign rule and brutally suppressed Filipino resistance. In 1935, President Roosevelt proclaimed the Philippines a constitutional commonwealth and established an eleven-year timeline for the country to transition into full independence. The Filipino people, it seemed, were so close to achieving the independence they had long craved.

The farewells were still difficult. Dorothy stood at the train station in Los Angeles with her parents, sister, and infant nephew. Her brother-in-law was absent due to work, but he sent a message for "Dixie" to have a good time.

"Tell him I intend to!" Dorothy told her sister optimistically.

Around 6:00 AM, the loudspeaker in the hospital at Cavite crackled. A slight static popped, and everyone paused to hear the announcement. "Hear this," a man's voice thundered. "Pearl Harbor has been bombed."

The patients had mixed reactions. Men eligible for discharge were eager to give the Japanese a good pounding. They anticipated the fight would be fast and easy. For the patients with broken limbs, there was a helpless feeling of vulnerability. They were marooned on their backs with cast-covered limbs suspended in the air. If the hospital was hit, they were tethered in place, unable to run or even roll under the bed for protection.

An attack on the hospital was a terrifying possibility. The Empire of Japan had signed but did not ratify the Third Geneva Convention, which meant they never agreed hospitals were off limits. And the empire had already violated the Hague Convention of 1907—which it once pledged to uphold—by bombing Pearl Harbor without first declaring war or issuing a warning. The navy nurses were only several hours into the conflict and they already knew they weren't dealing with an honorable enemy. The 150-bed hospital needed to be emptied and prepared to receive causalities.

Patients stood single file with charts in hand. A physician swiftly reviewed each case, flipping through the chart and deciding if discharge papers were indeed appropriate. Men were classified as "ambulatory" and ready for discharge or as a "no-go" who required evacuation. Dorothy felt concerned as men assured the physician they would continue to take their medicines. Others promised to keep their bandages clean or not put too much weight on a healing sprain.

Dorothy found that most able-bodied men were anxious to leave the hospital. The sailors wanted to return to their assignments, and the civilians needed to get home to their families. But the men with broken limbs, severe infections, diseases, or undiagnosed conditions had no way of escaping a label of "no-go." They were sent back to their beds with a sense of vulnerability.

Dorothy followed a physician as he worked his way down the ward, writing discharge or transfer papers for the patients still in bed. At the end of the row, a sailor recently released from the iron lung asked to be discharged. Of all the nurses, Dorothy spent the most time tending to the iron lung patients. She knew the man's condition and felt he was too unstable for discharge. Until just a few days earlier, he had relied on the pressurized machine to force his weak lungs to breathe. The physician neglected to consult her opinion, and she cringed as he signed discharge papers.

A jittery current streamed through the wards as rumors heightened the anxiety. One man repeated how he heard the Japanese had blasted the California coast. Dorothy immediately thought of her family. What if her parents were injured by a bomb? Were her sister, brother-in-law, and nephew safe?

The Japanese did not reach California. The threat was much closer to Dorothy. The Japanese military turned its attention toward the Philippines that morning and bombed Camp John Hay, an army outpost located in the mountains. The attacking planes dropped more than 128 bombs. Thirty-seven casualties were rushed to the tiny hospital, where only two nurses and one surgeon were on duty. War had indeed come to the Philippines—the navy nurses at Cavite just didn't know it yet.

Outside the hospital, sailors stacked sandbags around the building. Inside, the nurses were submerged in the hospital's liquidation. By 10:30 AM, most patients had received either discharge or transfer orders. The discharged men simply walked out the front door with their papers. The transfers were far more complicated. Other military hospitals were in the midst of their own evacuations and not inclined to add to their own patient census. Dorothy noticed her superiors seemed flustered. Nurse Margaret "Peg" Nash passed Dorothy and whispered how Chief Nurse Cobb had given her contradicting assignments and then seemed irritated when nothing was completed.

Peg was a recent transfer from the naval base in Guam. The petite nurse had been assisting in surgery when she received urgent instructions to step away from the operating table and prepare for immediate transfer to the Philippines. The unexpected transfer ripped her away from her fiancé, Edwin. The couple planned for Edwin to take leave in February 1942 and marry Peg in the Philippines. Until then, Peg was assigned to Ward C with Dorothy.

Their ward was a mess. Fifty sailors and marines had already received discharge papers and left behind rumpled beds with soiled linens. Dorothy was keen to order her corpsmen* to replace the bedding so that the ward could be sterilized. But it was near lunchtime, and the other nurses urged her to return to the nurses' quarters for a meal.

Dorothy and the nurses had just sat down when the air raid siren began to blare. The nurses continued munching as they listened to the urgent wail. A few hours earlier, the siren was briefly tested and then silenced. Was it another drill? Chief Nurse Cobb brusquely directly her nurses to take shelter underneath the quarters.

The nurses looked at her in disbelief. She really wanted them to go under the building and sit in the dirt wearing their all-white uniforms? Cobb's quiet irritation made it clear that yes, she did expect her nurses to sit in the dirt. She assured them a more suitable uniform was on order. Until then, they needed to take shelter. The women obediently filed past Cobb and headed underneath the building. They flicked on their flashlights and sat on the ground, trying to tug at their skirts so the dirt didn't smear against their bare thighs.

---

* A corpsman is an enlisted man assigned to assist dentists, nurses, pharmacists, and physicians.

To the nurses, it felt like another drill. They did not know that Clark Field, an army air base about seventy miles away, was under assault. The Japanese air force had flown nighttime reconnaissance missions and they knew where to find the airfields. On the runway, refueling planes were exposed. It was terrible timing for the United States and only a few of the men caught on the tarmac survived. By the time Dorothy and the other nurses emerged into the sunlight, the Japanese army had killed eighty people, injured civilians, and succeeded in annihilating the US Army's Far East air force. The nurses did not know how easy it would be for the Japanese to come for the navy. They only had to pick the day.

After the all clear, Chief Nurse Laura Cobb called the women into the living room for a meeting. Two nurses were being transferred to Sternberg, a nearby army hospital, along with a team of corpsmen and two doctors. She asked for two volunteers. Neither Dorothy nor nurse Carrie Edwina Todd, known as Edwina, offered to go. Both women had orders to return to the United States on January 1, 1942. They preferred to finish their last few weeks in the Philippines in their familiar home. The other women remained silent as well. They instinctively feared the unknown.

Nurse Mary Frances Chapman eventually volunteered. Earlier in the year, she had requested an extension so she could stay with her fiancé in the Philippines. Now that a wedding date was set, her resignation was submitted and her passage home was booked. She anticipated she would not be part of any hostilities for long.

Mary urged her good friend nurse Ann Bernatitus to join her at Sternberg. Ann wasn't interested in the idea. Neither were the other nurses. What if they agreed and then something terrible happened? They didn't want to make a decision they might later regret.

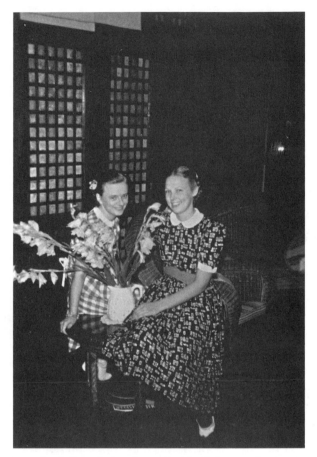

Dorothy Still and C. Edwina Todd off duty at Cavite, in civilian clothes. The nurses were advised to pack plenty of party dresses for their time at Cavite. *Courtesy of Bureau of Medicine and Surgery*

Chief Cobb did not have time for hesitation. "Who is going to volunteer?" she asked. Cobb continued to repeat her question as the women averted their eyes.

Ann resented that Mary had associated her name with the transfer. It felt as though everyone now assumed the spot should go to her. "Why don't you make us draw straws?" she suggested, hoping she would not draw the short stick.

Cobb left the room and returned with long applicator sticks topped with cotton swabs. Nurse Goldia O'Haver drew the first stick. It was clearly the longest of the bunch and she knew she was safe. Cobb walked over to Ann. She selected a cotton tip and pulled out the attached stick. It was the shortest one—Ann was going to Sternberg after all. The nurses roared with laughter. Ann sourly held up the short stick as another nurse gave her a reassuring pat on the back.

Cobb waited for her nurses to settle themselves. She had more business to address. Cobb pulled out a stack of sailors' uniforms—work shirts and dark blue dungarees. The women again shrieked with laughter. The work shirts weren't so problematic, but the dungaree pants were meant for a sailor's physique. The pants typically sat comfortably on a man's narrow pelvis but came up short on a woman's round hips. The women chortled at the thought of wearing the ill-fitted pants instead of a nurse's uniform. A few of the nurses humored the other women by pulling on the dungarees and showing off the ridiculous fit.

"I'd die before I wore those!" Peg Nash announced to the group.

Chief Nurse Cobb bristled. She thought she'd done everyone a favor when she accepted the uniforms from a supply officer. She curtly reminded her nurses that the dungarees might be helpful. Until they received uniform replacements, they had to tolerate the men's pants. As their dusty dresses indicated, white simply wouldn't do in wartime. Cobb ordered each nurse to pack several sets in her trunk and then return to the hospital to prepare the wards and the surgical suites.

Dorothy found the work steadied her. The corpsmen stripped and remade the beds with fresh linen. They pulled and tugged each bed frame until the rows were properly spaced. They brought in extra blankets, folded them, and neatly set them aside. The nurses rolled and readied bandages. They distilled gallons of water and prepared saline solutions. They filled IV bags and saw that the bedside trays were set with water pitchers, drinking glasses, stirs, and gauze. The nurses inventoried the medical lockers. They turned out labels, refilled bottles, and made sure stoppers were properly plugged. Chief Nurse Cobb readied the opioids in case patients presented with substantial injuries that required morphine. Dorothy made sure her ward received the plasma she ordered as well as the intravenous sets. The pristine placement gave Dorothy a sense of security. If Cavite was attacked, the nurses were ready to respond.

When Dorothy woke on Tuesday morning, she learned the United States and its allies had declared war on the Empire of Japan. Back in the hospital, the medical personnel continued to evacuate the "no-gos." Dorothy listened uneasily to the sounds of Ward C. Patients chatted casually with each other as they awaited transfer papers. Dorothy thought it sounded more like a social gathering than a hospital in the midst of an evacuation. If she closed her eyes, she could have imagined herself back at the Jai Alai Building* wearing a party dress and heading into a dance on an officer's arm. She knew all of that was now over. Before bed the previous night, she'd packed her party dresses into a trunk along with her other clothes, jewelry, and books. She placed her white uniforms on the top.

Transfer and movement were on her mind as she walked out of the ward and headed into the nurses' office. She took a seat at a table. She had a stack of prescriptions to sort through as well as supply requisition forms and discharge papers. Naval procedure demanded that every element of patient care be documented. Dorothy never snubbed procedure, but the pressure of the evacuation made the multiple sets of paperwork seem like a hindrance.

---

* Jai alai is a racquet sport. The Jai Alai Building was a club with courts for the game as well as banquet halls and dining rooms.

Dorothy was soon interrupted with updates about Pearl Harbor. There were reports that all eight battleships in the harbor were sunk. Almost two hundred vessels were hit, including cruisers, destroyers, and minelayers.* The descriptions of the destruction made Dorothy feel vulnerable. Were they next? How could the United States defend itself if the fleet was incapacitated?

Details about the casualties also gave her pause. Thousands of people were killed or injured—almost all of them sailors. About 60 percent of patients were severely burned, with first- or second-degree burns on up to 80 percent of their bodies. There were also supply complications, and the hospital at Pearl Harbor ran short of plasma and tannic acid. The acid was crucial—compresses were soaked in the precious solution and then pressed on scorched flesh.

Dorothy's eyes widened as she listened to the casualty reports and the hospital's struggle to respond. Perhaps the enemy was fiercer and more prepared than she once assumed.

---

* A minelayer plants mines in the open water.

2

Oh My God,
This Is Really War

TWO AIR RAID sirens interrupted Dorothy's overnight hours. Twice she sprang from her bed and into the makeshift shelter beneath the nurses' quarters. Both disruptions were false alarms that fatigued everyone. Wednesday morning was quiet, and people were sluggish. Dorothy and the other nurses wore the dungarees and work shirts that Chief Nurse Cobb provided. The "suitable alternatives" had yet to arrive, and the nurses were trying to adjust to the awkwardness of wearing men's clothing. They tugged at the waist and adjusted the folds of fabric. Nurse Peg was good humored as her fellow nurses reminded her she swore she'd die before she wore dungarees.

The ward was empty, and the stillness made Dorothy uncomfortable. She passed the morning shift in the nurses' office, going over paperwork and chatting with corpsmen who leaned casually on the doorframe and complained of their exhaustion. Around noon, Dorothy walked back to the nurses' quarters for lunch.

Dorothy sat with the other women in their dining room. One of the women spread the *Manila Tribune* on the table. The front-page story provided tips on how citizens should protect themselves if bombs pounded the city. The same article also asked readers to remain calm and not panic when under attack.

The nurses were not sure what to think. Their fleet was not equipped for battle. Sailors in the naval yard were working furiously to repair ships, submarines, and destroyers. But there was so much that needed to be done. One minesweeper still had disassembled engine parts. The largest ship in the yard was in the process of being converted from a merchant vessel to a destroyer. A few vessels only required fuel, but several were tied together, which made a quick escape difficult.

The morning's headlines about the Pearl Harbor attack felt like an ominous warning. Dorothy offered assurances the fleet could mobilize quickly and respond to any assault. "Don't worry," Dorothy said between forkfuls. As she ate, she tried to convince herself that her confidence in the fleet was warranted.

And then the air raid warning sounded. The wailing siren blared like a wave, starting low with a short crescendo to a full blast and then fading as a second wave began. The nurses picked up their plates and stood up from the table. All the other air raids had been false alarms, and no one wanted to miss a meal. Taking their food with them, they hurried outside, past the sandbags and underneath the building.

The hesitant conversation was replaced with a new, more confident chatter. The women rationalized that Pearl Harbor was surprised by the attack. The US Navy at Cavite was warned and ready. Several of the nurses even suggested it would be a quick fight. After all, they justified, Japan was a much smaller country. Mary Rose reminded everyone that Japan wasn't even the size of her home state of South Dakota. Several nurses nodded in agreement as they continued eating their lunch. Cavite, they decided, was going to be the US Armed Forces' retribution for Pearl Harbor.

Two cooks stood near the entrance to the shelter. They saw a formation of Japanese planes speeding in from the north, across Manila Bay. "Here they come!" they yelled.

The nurses braced for the attack, but the formation flew past them high and fast. Directly across the peninsula, an antiaircraft battery fired at the enemy. The nurses heard the gunfire and Dorothy felt assured. She was confident the navy was knocking down planes and forcing the Japanese to retreat.

Dorothy did not know the planes soared at twenty-four thousand feet and the battery's shells didn't come close to hitting the formation. The shells fruitlessly exploded and left behind balloons of black smoke that lingered in the air and advertised the failure. The formation passed without attacking, circled, and then turned back toward the peninsula. Another battery fired in defense, and the men were frantic when their firepower again failed to reach the attackers.

Then the bombs hit, and the nurses jolted from the concussion. Dorothy pulled her knees to her chest and clenched, knowing they would die if the nurses' quarters took a direct hit. With each thundering blast, she wondered if the next bomb would detonate on top of them. The drone of the planes briefly dissipated as the formation circled back over the bay. The nurses heard the chugging of machine gun fire from the antiaircraft batteries and the response from enemy planes. The ground quaked as the next wave of bombs rained on the small peninsula.

In their shelter, the nurses smelled the destruction they had yet to see. The chemicals used in the bombs left behind a stench that resembled burning rubber. The odor mixed with the flames streaming from the demolition. Nurse Peg pulled out her rosary and began moving her quivering hands through the beads. Dorothy watched her lips move: *Holy Mary, Mother of God, pray for us sinners, now and at the hour of our death.* Mary Rose gripped her own rosary, pressing her fingers against the beads and then the chain. *As it was in the beginning is now, and ever shall be, world without end.*

Dorothy looked around the shelter at the other nurses. Seeing the terror on their faces reinforced her own fear. Edwina took off her glasses, as if she didn't want to witness any of the destruction. She looked over and smiled weakly in Dorothy's direction. Dietitian Bertha was so terrified she went into the fight-or-flight response. The color drained from her face, which suggested she was desperate to flee, but she managed a smile in Dorothy's direction. Dorothy's good friend Eldene Paige quietly quivered. It was Eldene's twenty-eighth birthday, and her shaking hands indicated she worried it might be her last. All the women were trembling, but they did not cry. No one hyperventilated or panicked. They sat quietly, trading the occasional comforting smile with each other.

After almost an hour, dense smoke darkened the sky and blocked the attackers from identifying their targets. The Japanese moved on. Soon the nurses heard the all-clear siren. It was their signal to get to the hospital and nurse the wounded.

Chief Cobb looked at the eleven women huddled and shaking before her. "No point in waiting any longer," she ordered.

Dorothy climbed past the sandbags and surfaced from underneath the nurses' quarters. She was finally able to glimpse everything she'd heard for the past hour. Cavite was ringed in fire. A wall of flames burned in the yard and black plumes of smoke surged into the sky. Across the bay, Manila was ablaze. The Japanese bombers had hit civilian targets too.

Chief Nurse Cobb yelled for the women to run. *Move, go, hurry!* Dorothy began sprinting. From a block away, she saw the hospital was still standing. She raced toward the door, passing shredded structures

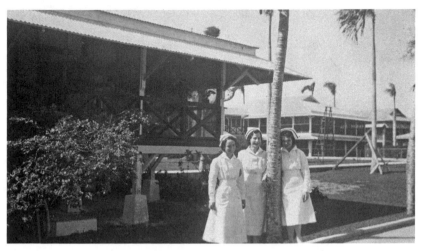

Eldene Paige, Laura Cobb, and Peg Nash at Cavite before the war. During the bombing, the nurses hid underneath their dormitory, which was similar to the one seen in the background. *Courtesy of Bureau of Medicine and Surgery*

and downed trees. Cavite, she realized, had not been the United States' chance for retribution. The United States hadn't won the battle, and war with Japan would not be a quick fight.

Dorothy ran up the hospital's circular drive and joined the turmoil. Injured and unconscious men were already inside, brought by glassy-eyed survivors who swiftly dumped the bodies and rushed to help others. Casualties were arriving so quickly that corpsmen placed them in any available bed. Dorothy panted as she hurried to Ward C with Peg. They paused at the doorway, stunned by the astounding display of injured men.

"Oh my God, this is really war," Peg gasped.

Dorothy scanned the ward. The corpsmen were hauling in men with gashes, severe dislocations, head injuries, and missing limbs. Dorothy saw compound fractures with shattered bones bursting through the skin. Some patients seemed to have all their muscles pouring from a split in their arm or leg. Men with paralyzing dislocations were dragged into the ward. Arms and legs bent in unnatural ways. Dorothy glimpsed broken hips that jutted the leg out to the side and splintered knees that pushed the lower leg into a ninety-degree angle. Broken ankles twisted feet in the wrong direction, and disjointed shoulders made arms hang helplessly. Many of the patients with broken bones or dislocated joints urged the nurses to tend to others with more serious injuries. Dorothy and Peg moved on to patients with uncontrollable bleeding from deep lacerations.

And then the burn victims arrived. One singed man gasped about the lock on the naval yard. Men were trapped, he told Dorothy. He'd heard them screaming as they burned to death. Dorothy nodded as she gave the man a shot of morphine. She needed water to cool his skin, but she had to triage other casualties. There were men with second-degree burns that were red, swollen, and seething with blisters. Others had profound, third-degree burns that penetrated past the skin and into the deeper tissues. Dorothy saw skin that was charred black from flames, as well as scalded white skin already shedding the outer layer.

The ward filled with sounds of agony. Men moaned and whimpered. They screamed and wept. One man was missing his arm. The nerves that ran down his arm were ripped from his spinal cord, leaving only a mutilated stump with frayed endings. Dorothy approached the man with a shot of morphine. She quickly injected a quarter of a grain of morphine under his skin. He would have an agonizing ten minutes until the morphine blurred his pain. It was a heavy dose and Dorothy expected it to last for up to four hours. The surgeons, if they were able to get to him, could not do much for the man, other than clean and stitch the wound.

There were patients with limbs hanging on by one stubborn ligament. The bones, muscles, and nerves were completely severed, and Dorothy knew amputation was inevitable. She bent over a patient with a nearly severed leg, pushing down on the syringe and watching the morphine inject. Then she moved on to the next patient.

She inspected patients with deep gashes. As she injected the morphine, the men panted and cried to Dorothy, wanting to tell her what happened. Several were in shock, repeatedly telling Dorothy how they tried to fire back. In their minds, the men were still with their battery, aiming their arms toward the sky and helplessly watching their defense fail.

Dorothy froze when one of the sailors revealed how the medical dispensary was hit. Just before the bombing, the sailor had carried an injured friend to the dispensary for help. The sailor hurried down the road and wasn't far when he saw a bomb obliterate the building. Dorothy immediately thought of the medical personnel who were at the dispensary. *My boys*, she thought to herself. *My brothers*. She assured herself they were safe. It was the only way she could carry on.

Dorothy had to keep nursing. She could not stop. The wards faced a deluge of casualties, and everything was further strained by the power outage. The power plant, the nurses learned, was hit first and ignited on impact. The officer in charge ordered the plant to shut down so an explosion would not annihilate the peninsula. In the naval yard, fire crews battled the spreading inferno without power. They circled the ammunition depot and fought back the blazes that threatened to set off the combustibles inside.

And at the hospital, the medical corps struggled without electricity. The surgery was problematically located on the third floor. The elevators were dead, and corpsmen arduously carried wounded men up the stairs. The power outage brought other crises. The water boiler couldn't produce steam, which meant sterilizing instruments was no longer an option. A doctor issued a directive that needles could be replaced, but syringes had to be reused between patients. And if the supply of sterile needles ran out, then the nurses knew what they had to do.

Dorothy stiffened as she saw two soot-covered corpsmen lift a dead man from a bed and head toward the morgue. Another set of soiled corpsmen heaved a waiting patient off the floor and placed him on the fouled bed. Dorothy knew it was impossible to change the linens between patients, but it sickened her to think of the possible infections they faced.

There was no time to complain, and Dorothy continued to work. She moved from one patient to the next, firmly pushing a needle under the skin and injecting morphine. She wrapped tourniquets around heavily bleeding wounds or pressed down with a bandage. She felt for pulses on lifeless bodies and ordered for the dead to be taken to the morgue.

Dorothy bent over patients with sterile bandages and set out to clean wounds. As she rinsed away oil and blood, she often found the injury was much deeper than it appeared. At times, she suspected that a patient was hemorrhaging internally. Dorothy progressed through the crowd, trying to make sure that every man was triaged. But the casualties kept coming, and civilians soon arrived on the hospital's front lawn. Many were burned or unresponsive, and they were carried by family members on makeshift stretchers. Locals used blankets, carpets, and even doors to bring bombing victims to the hospital.

People of all ages filled the ward. Dorothy saw dazed grandmothers sitting next to small children on the floor, blotting their tears and mourning dead family members. Dorothy recognized one elderly woman as a relative of the nurses' cook. Only a few hours earlier, he'd prepared the lunch they'd brought into the shelter. When the air raid started, he tried to ride his bicycle home to be with his family. The older woman told Dorothy the cook died on his way home.

Dorothy blinked back tears. She was upset about the cook and sick about the medical personnel in the dispensary. And she was devastated by the pain and suffering that surrounded her. She walked away from the older woman, forcing herself to focus. The ward was now so choked with casualties that she stumbled between patients. The cots that had once been neatly aligned were in disarray, and some mattresses were shared by multiple patients. Latecomers were reduced to lying on the floor or sitting painfully upright in chairs. The hospital was several hundred patients over capacity.

The ward descended into chaos, with only two nurses, Dorothy and Peg, to tend to all the wounded. Corpsmen tried to help, but there was a complete lack of communication as to which patients had yet to be seen. Dorothy and Peg soon lost track of who had received attention and who still needed a dose of morphine. Dorothy decided to take charge. She asked a corpsman for anything that would allow her to chart. He returned with a box of tags from the morgue. Dorothy did not have time to argue the morbid inappropriateness of the tags. She took the box and began attaching the tags to the wrists of patients who had been triaged. Dorothy inched through the crowded ward, kneeling next to each patient and pulling a tag onto his or her wrist.

She knelt down next to an unconscious sailor and pulled up the dog tag from around his neck, transferring the information onto a morgue tag—name, serial number, and blood type—and scribbled a brief note on his condition. She attached the tag to his wrist and moved to the next man. Reading his dog tag, she asked him if he'd had morphine yet. She made it a point to call him by his name. These patients, she realized, were alone. The brief interaction they shared was a powerful assurance that someone was watching over them.

The sailor looked into Dorothy's hazel eyes and knew he could trust her. He was traumatized and began crying. "You can't believe what it was like," he told her.

Dorothy wiped the tears from his dirty cheeks. She told him that she was getting a good sense of what happened. "I'll be back to check on you again," she promised.

Dorothy had to help others. All the patients had stories they wanted to tell her. She listened and soothed one sailor as he described dragging his friend to the hospital. Dorothy tried to hear her patients through the shrill of suffering. Adults were in hysterics. Children were sobbing. Frightened babies wailed. Patients begged for help. There was also a pungent smell to the room—a stench of burned skin, blood, oil, urine, and feces. The odor was a reminder that Dorothy was no longer in a regular hospital. She was nursing under fire.

A little boy asked for a glass of water. Dorothy stood over him and promised to return as soon as she had a chance. She was torn away by oozing burns and hyperventilating patients. The little boy repeated his request to Peg, but she also had other traumas to address first. There were new arrivals who badly needed morphine and evaluation. Peg eventually found a moment to fill a glass with water. She returned to the boy and tried to offer it to him. He didn't respond. Peg grabbed his wrist and pressed three fingers on the artery. She counted silently to herself, waiting to feel a pulsation.

The next time Peg passed Dorothy, she told her the little boy had died. Dorothy admitted he'd asked her for water, but she was tied up with more pressing patients. Neither woman realized the boy was in the last moments of his life. Even if they had known, there wasn't much they could have done for him. There were hundreds of other patients, and most were screaming in agony. They couldn't have sat with the boy or held him while he passed. The child died alone.

Peg quietly wondered if it would be best if the Japanese planes returned, dropped a bomb, and ended all the suffering. The patients who would not survive were in the midst of an excruciating end. And the survivors would be forever traumatized by their injuries as well as the agony they witnessed. Dorothy thought the only ones in the ward who had any peace were those who were already dead.

3

Everything Under Control

CHIEF NURSE LAURA Cobb was being pulled in every direction. Nurses in the wards were asking for help. The corpsmen wanted direction. The surgical teams needed her. Cobb rotated between the wards and the surgery, maintaining the appearance of a calm demeanor she likely did not feel. Cobb strode into Ward C, looking for either Dorothy or Peg. She made note of the makeshift tags Dorothy had placed on patients' wrists. Morbid, yes, but an improvement on the other wards' methods. One ward was marking foreheads with lipstick to indicate the patient was triaged. At least they were improvising solutions. Cobb now needed the nurses to establish a system, however crude, for getting patients up to the third-floor surgical suites.

"Line them up," Cobb ordered Peg.

Peg and Dorothy directed the corpsmen to create a line of patients who needed surgery. The line was adjusted to prioritize more critical patients. A patient with gaping torso wounds, the women explained, should be placed ahead of a sailor with a missing foot—assuming the new amputee's bleeding was controlled and he only required stitching.

A line began to form, first in the hallways outside the surgical suites. As the hallways filled, the corpsmen balanced bodies on the stair risers and plunked patients on the landings. It was a wretched, dismayed queue. Patients sat in a morphine-induced haze, sometimes oblivious to the agonized howling around them. Surgeons in blood-stained gowns sporadically appeared to assess the misery. At their instruction, corpsmen scooped critical patients from the middle or the back of the line and carried them into surgery. The surgeons also performed straightforward procedures on the staircase, such as snipping off the lone ligament that attached a hand to a wrist. The severed limb was handed to a corpsman to toss into a growing heap of detached fingers, hands, feet, arms, and legs.

Nurse anesthetist Susie Pitcher sedated patients in the surgery. With the electricity out, nurse Goldia O'Haver rinsed instruments in Lysol and rushed them to the surgeons. The surgical team improvised and tried to fight against the despair. But they flailed in the chaos. The floor was slick from spilled bodily fluids, and they battled to stay upright. Blood saturated their gowns and soaked through to their skin. The team rotated through patients, trying to rouse life from bodies condemned to die.

Downstairs, dietitian Bertha Evans was reassigned from her kitchen duties to perform triage in the wards. She worked with a feeling of detachment. Everything felt surreal to Bertha, as if it were happening to someone else and she was an observer, like a patron at the cinema watching a newsreel before the main feature.

Bertha approached unconscious patients and lifted their wrists. Nurses did not carry stethoscopes and instead felt for a pulse to determine whether a patient was still alive. Bertha failed to find a pulse for one unconscious sailor. He did not appear to be breathing and his skin was cold and clammy. She wasn't certain, and she called Peg over for a second opinion.

"Peg," Bertha asked. "See if you can get a pulse on this fellow."

Peg took the man's wrist and pressed down with her fingers. She did not feel a heartbeat. She moved her fingers to his neck and placed her finger on his carotid artery. Nothing.

"I guess he's expired," Peg confirmed.

Bertha flagged down a corpsman. He lifted the body onto a gurney, covered him with a sheet, and wheeled the patient toward the morgue. As the gurney left the ward, the movement jarred the patient awake. He sat up suddenly. "Where am I?" he demanded.

The corpsman sulkily reported the incident to Peg and Bertha. It had given him a fright, as if he had seen a body rise from the dead. The nurses realized the man had been in circulatory shock, which caused low blood pressure and slowed his pulse so significantly that his heartbeat was undetectable without a stethoscope. The shock also made his skin cold and moist, as if he had been dead for several hours. Peg and Bertha felt relief the patient was alive and most likely to survive his ordeal. For a moment, the incident almost struck them as funny, as if a practical joke had been played on the corpsman.

The respite was fleeting. People were dying. In the wards, patients perished from blood loss. Others had internal bruising on their organs caused by the impact of the explosions. Such injuries could be invisible, with the patient capable of speaking lucidly about his ordeal. When the nurses came back to check, they might find the patient blankly staring at a world he had already exited.

Ward C became sadly quieter as the afternoon progressed. Many of the casualties died and were transferred to the morgue. Stable patients were evacuated from the hospital to a makeshift accommodation. In the early evening, Dorothy found time to update the paperwork. These records were crucial, providing documentation as to who was injured and who had died. Back in the States, there were widows whose survivors' benefits depended on these reports, because the navy stopped paychecks for men missing in action.

Peg and Dorothy sat together, jotting notes. With the power out, they worked in the dim light of kerosene lamps and flashlights. The nurses had initially been concerned about adhering to blackout orders and attempted to work in the dark. One of the captains, R. G. Davis, issued a directive for the lights to remain on while the hospital was liquidated. Captain Davis chose not to disclose that he had received a terrifying warning from the Japanese military. The hospital had thirty-six hours to evacuate or they would be bombed. The navy wanted the hospital emptied before dawn.

Dorothy put down her pencil and decided to round the ward. Most of the patients were sedated or sleeping, but one called for her softly when she passed.

"Nurse," the sailor summoned weakly.

Dorothy approached the bed, picked up the man's arm, and read his tag.

"Are you having trouble going to sleep?" she whispered, careful not to wake the other patients. She offered him a sip of water to moisten his mouth. He declined. He just wanted to talk.

"I'm going to die," the sailor told Dorothy with a calm voice, as if he were stating any other fact. Dorothy paused and studied the young man. He was lucid. He did not seem to be in distress.

Dorothy assured the sailor he had been through a lot and was likely in shock. She wiped his face with a moist cloth. She felt his pulse and told him he would be fine.

"It's true," the sailor repeated. "I'm going to die."

Dorothy encouraged the man not to think negatively. The next day would be better. "Not for me," the sailor countered. He explained how a surgeon had told a nurse there was no use trying to stitch him up. He'd be dead before the night was over.

His story struck Dorothy as amiss. It was standard practice at the time not to disclose a patient's prognosis. The medical community considered the information potentially damaging to a patient's will to live. But the day had been unlike any other, and it was possible the surgeon had let it slip in the rush. Dorothy suggested that the sailor misunderstood. She tried to be positive and told him not to worry.

The sailor insisted he knew he was in his final hours. He'd also heard the surgeon order the nurse to put on heavy dressings and send him to the ward to die. "See for yourself," he offered.

Dorothy peeled back his covers. Underneath, there was a rubber sheet as well as a surgical warming blanket. The blanket was doubled up, and both layers were saturated with blood and serum. Dorothy lifted the blanket and was punched by the stench of blood and bowels. She suppressed the urge to retch. The sailor's torso was indeed gravely damaged by a blast. The surface flesh peeled from his body. No muscles, tendons, fat, or skin remained. His intestines were exposed, and Dorothy saw fecal matter oozing from the battered bowels. The surgeon was correct. The patient didn't have any remaining skin to stitch. Infection would soon take hold, and Dorothy expected the sailor would die within the next few days. She wished the surgeon had handled the diagnosis with more delicacy.

The quiet and darkness of the ward gave Dorothy a moment to reflect on the man's unique misery. Other patients were also in their final hours of life. But they were unconscious or unaware that their lives were dimming. This sailor knew he was dying. He was awake and trying to make sense of the violent ending to his short life. Dorothy wanted to mitigate his mental anguish. "You must have misunderstood," she lied.

Dorothy held both of the sailor's hands and asked if he was in any pain. He said he was not, and she promised she'd return to check on him. She continued down the row, looking to see who was awake or restless. She returned to the paperwork and attempted to focus on the records. Her mind kept drifting back to the patient.

Dorothy decided to check on him. She'd let him talk some more. Or help him write a letter home to his parents or sweetheart. She turned down the aisle and was surprised by the empty bed. She asked a corpsman if he knew anything about the patient. The corpsman wearily explained that the man had been pronounced dead within the last ten minutes and his body had already been brought to the morgue. Dorothy looked down at the empty bed and felt in danger of losing control of her emotions. She could not wake the patients or scare them with her sobbing. She pushed past the corpsman and hurried from the ward.

Dorothy wept outside the hospital. The humid air reeked of explosives and small fires continued to burn in the distance. Dorothy chided herself for not returning to the patient sooner. She thought of all the things she should have done to ease his suffering and then unfairly thought of herself as a coward. But there was no guidance in the *Navy Hospital Corps Handbook* on how to handle an onslaught of hundreds of dying patients. There was no formal procedure for comforting a lucid man who was in the final moments of his life.

Dorothy was traumatized. She had seen so much agony in the past eight hours that she was powerless to alleviate. They lacked supplies, space, sanitation, and staff. At times, she had only a shot of morphine and a comforting pat on the hand to offer to a whimpering patient. Dorothy took a few deep breaths and sniffled. The memories of mutilated bodies and screaming patients stirred up in her mind. She started to cry again, which felt frustrating. Her tears were one more thing she could not control.

She untucked her work shirt and patted her face dry, then smoothed her shirt underneath the dungarees and took a deep breath before heading back into the ward. Dorothy passed Peg as she hovered over a stack of records. They shared a comforting glance. Peg knew

Dorothy had been sobbing. She also knew her friend did not wish to discuss it. Peg instead encouraged Dorothy to go to the kitchen for a sandwich and a cup of a coffee.

Most of the surgeons were still operating, but a few doctors and corpsmen were in the kitchen. The men were seeking relief from the ordeal and joked about wanting a stiff drink. One corpsman had the room laughing when he told about a corpse sitting upright in the morgue and demanding a glass of water. It was another case of circulatory shock that startled an unsuspecting corpsman. Dorothy sipped her coffee and listened to their banter. The lights were dim, and she hoped no one could see her red eyes.

———————

Dorothy stood on the dock with nurse Mary Rose Harrington. Both women were dazed and exhausted. It was just after midnight on Thursday morning, and after almost twelve hours of nonstop nursing, Dorothy's remaining assignment was to wait for a transport boat. In the quiet, she realized she was numb. Everything had happened so quickly—the bombing, the influx of casualties, and the subsequent hours of death and despair. Now none of it felt real.

She thought of the comfortable routine she'd enjoyed at Cavite for almost two years. Every morning, she woke in her private room in the nurses' quarters. She went down to the dining room and ate breakfast provided by the domestic staff. She dressed in the standard uniform and walked to the hospital, past the rippling palm trees and scurrying geckos. Now the place in which she'd lived for the past two years had suddenly ceased to exist. It was too much for her mind to accept, and she stood on the dock with Mary Rose, not quite denying the destruction but unable to fully comprehend the loss.

A patrol torpedo boat soon approached. The vessel resembled a speedboat, but it was massive, about the length of two city buses.

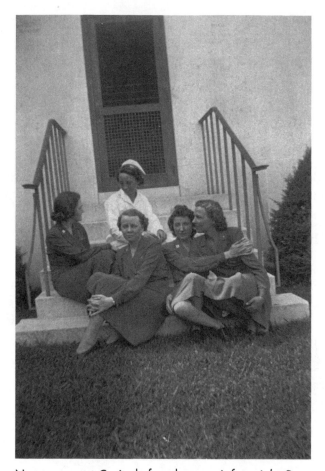

Navy nurses at Cavite before the war. *Left to right:* Peg
Nash, Eldene Paige *(on step above)*, Goldia O'Haver,
Helen Gorzelanski, and Dorothy Still. *Courtesy of Bureau
of Medicine and Surgery*

The boat was designed to launch torpedoes at enemy vessels and then
race away at speeds of up to fifty miles per hour. Dorothy had never
been on such a boat and marveled at the engineering. She wondered
how an enormous vessel moved so swiftly. One of the sailors revealed
that the bottom of the boat lacked any armor. The hull was really
plywood, which was why it was so light and fast.

Dorothy's admiration dissolved into vulnerability. They were under attack and she was being transported on an unarmored boat? She climbed aboard, knowing she had no option but to follow the evacuation orders. She could not refuse and demand a land transport. She was due in Manila. The army and navy were combining surgical efforts. Nurses were being divided into groups and sent to military and civilian hospitals. In the heart of Manila, the Jai Alai Building was being converted into a surgery. Dorothy was assigned there, along with nurse anesthetist Susie Pitcher.

The midnight air was cool, and the sailors suggested Dorothy and Mary Rose would be more comfortable below deck. Mary Rose accepted the invitation, but Dorothy wanted a broad view of the yard. She stood near the front of the vessel as it pulled back from the dock and quietly slid along the coast. In the dark, Dorothy squinted at the outlines of various buildings, trying to determine which structures were still standing. A few flickering flames provided a dim illumination. She saw heaps of rubble where dormitories and supply buildings had once stood. The boat turned toward Manila and sped up. Dorothy watched as her former home was absorbed by darkness.

Dorothy looked down at her feet. Just weeks before, she'd stood on the same staircase at the Jai Alai Building in Manila. At the time, she had walked on plush red carpeting with her hand wrapped around an officer's arm. Now the carpeting was ripped up, and the building that had once hosted candlelight dinners was rapidly being transformed into a hospital. Workers replaced the lush drapes with blackout curtains and tucked ornate lobby furniture into storage. The corpsmen crammed empty cots into the massive jai alai courts and awaited the inevitable casualties.

Japan was certain to unleash another round of airstrikes on the Philippine capital. Every air raid siren was heeded. Three days had passed since the bombing on Cavite. The US newspapers reported the attack, but there was a lot of misinformation, including a rumor that Japanese planes had flown over Los Angeles during the overnight hours. Several of the other navy nurses, including Susie and Edwina, sent telegrams home to their families, letting them know they had survived the attack and they hoped all was well on the home front.

Dorothy thought of her parents in Long Beach. She wanted to send them a quick message. One afternoon, she received permission to walk to the Manila Hotel to send her parents a telegram. She stood for hours in a long line that snaked through the lobby. As she waited, she traded information with sailors she knew from Cavite, trying to learn which friends and acquaintances had survived the attack. When she finally reached the Western Union counter, she sent a bright message that revealed nothing of her ordeal. "CHRISTMAS GREETINGS," she wrote in all capital letters. "DON'T WORRY ABOUT ME. EVERYTHING UNDER CONTROL."

It was after 8:00 PM when Dorothy left the hotel. She stood outside the lobby, trying to summon the courage to step into the inky air. Manila was under blackout orders, and the darkness intimidated her. She did not want to walk the one mile back to the Jai Alai Building in the pitch black. There was a line of people waiting at the taxi stand, and Dorothy worried it would be several hours before she secured a ride.

Dorothy walked down the circular drive, heading toward the street. At the end of the drive, she recognized a military sedan. She approached the driver's open window and asked for a ride. She explained that she was a nurse with the surgical team at the Jai Alai. The chauffeur declined. Dejected, Dorothy walked away.

"Having a problem?" a voice asked.

Dorothy turned around and faced an army officer who emerged from the sedan. He was a tall man, about six feet, and past sixty years old. "You might say so," she replied. Dorothy explained that she was part of the surgical teams.

"Army nurse?" the officer interrupted.

"No, sir," Dorothy said. "Navy nurse."

The officer leaned down to the chauffeur and instructed him to take Dorothy wherever she needed to go. He briskly strode off. Relieved, Dorothy climbed into the back seat of the sedan. Who was that man? She wondered. And could the driver thank him on her behalf?

The driver agreed to pass along her message of gratitude. "That's General Douglas MacArthur," he said.

General MacArthur was finally out and about, which likely was a relief to his senior commanders in the Philippines. After the attack on Pearl Harbor, MacArthur had holed up in his luxury penthouse at the Manila Hotel. He made himself inaccessible to commanders seeking direction. Knocks on the door were ignored and the phone jarringly rang without answer. In the coming months, MacArthur gained a reputation for choosing the best hiding places for himself and then rarely emerging. The enlisted men called him "dugout Doug."

In his well-appointed penthouse, MacArthur received disturbing communication from his superiors in Washington, DC. President Franklin D. Roosevelt had met with Henry Stimson, the secretary of war, and two army generals, Dwight Eisenhower and George Marshal. Behind closed doors, they had admitted the United States was militarily weak. Although streams of motivated young men were lining up at recruitment offices, it would take months to train new troops and ship them to Europe or the South Pacific. And the United States was still woefully behind on producing the heavy machinery needed for battle.

To complicate matters, the United States was not alone in the fight against Axis powers. By mid-December, America was forming an alliance with China, France, Russia, and the United Kingdom. British prime minister Winston Churchill met in Washington with other Allied leaders on December 22 to discuss strategy. Churchill was pushing for a "Germany First" approach, envisioning a strategy in which Allied troops charged at Germany from every direction, effectively "closing the ring" around the country and strangling it into submission.

Roosevelt, however, knew that public sentiment in America favored revenge against Japan. The talks were friendly, but interests required alignment. Roosevelt had another reelection to consider and feared he would not fare well if Pearl Harbor was not properly avenged. But Roosevelt's options were limited. The United States was not battle ready. Within the day, Churchill received the president's assurance that the United States would focus on the European theater.

Both Roosevelt and Stimson actually confided to Churchill that they were already considering the Philippines to be a loss. Stimson coldly acknowledged that the "Europe First" strategy was effectively a death sentence for the US troops stationed in the Philippines. They were being abandoned by their country. "There are times when men have to die," Stimson said.

Was retreat an option? Some questioned whether the US forces should evacuate their troops and medical personnel. Military planners considered the Philippines indefensible, and they advocated for pulling out of the islands and heading to Australia to regroup. Naval commander Admiral Thomas C. Hart wanted to move south and guard Australia while the Allies built a defense. Hart had strongly disagreed with MacArthur, particularly during the summer of 1941 when the United States considered withdrawing from the Philippines and MacArthur optimistically advocated to remain. Hart had responded by sending much of his fleet to the Dutch East Indies* prior to the attack on Cavite.

General MacArthur soon learned Washington was not sending any reinforcements. Roosevelt's advisors did not think supply ships could evade the Japanese vessels that stalked the Philippine Sea. MacArthur was denied every request—ammunition, reserve troops, fresh battleships, minelayers, and torpedo boats. The United States was not sending fighter aircraft or attack bombers. Medicine and food supplies would not be replenished. MacArthur was completely on his own. Still, he rejected the possibility of retreat.

MacArthur pushed ahead with War Plan Orange, a combat strategy that had been devised several years earlier in the event that Japan attacked US interests in the South Pacific. The plan involved pulling out of Manila and heading to the nearby Bataan Peninsula as well as Corregidor, a well-positioned island in Manila Bay. The plan was well devised, but it was doomed. War Plan Orange required a steady replenishment of food, medicine, and artillery. Without such delivery, Japan would be able to close a ring around the Philippines and swiftly smother the resistance.

Admiral Hart wasn't lingering to watch the doomed defense. The Japanese successfully landed in the northern Philippine Islands and were pushing south toward the capital. Hart departed Manila on Christmas Day in a submarine destined for the Indies. The two remaining destroyers followed the next day. When Hart abandoned the Philippines, he also left behind injured and ill sailors, as well as the nurses who cared for them.

---

* Known today as Indonesia, the colonies that made up the Dutch East Indies were located about one thousand miles southwest of the Philippine Islands.

At the Jai Alai Building, Dorothy sat in an empty ward with nurse anesthetist Susie Pitcher, three surgeons, and about thirty corpsmen. The week had been quiet at the makeshift surgery. The civilians never realized the club had been turned into a hospital. After air raids, they brought their casualties to civilian or military hospitals. The ward's beds were empty, except for those occupied by lounging corpsmen.

The surgeons hunched over decks of cards, passing the quiet days with games that no longer amused. Dorothy played gin rummy, trying for hours to improve on the hand she was dealt. The game bore a strange resemblance to her current situation and she often became frustrated. In her anxiety, Dorothy peppered Susie with questions. When would the navy nurses receive their next orders? Would they be evacuated soon?

Susie seemed to cringe whenever Dorothy's nervous voice broke her concentration. The quiet was eerie, yes, but it was also a welcome break. Susie used the time to page through magazines and read novels. She did not want to speculate about the empty ward or the navy's next move. Susie's terse one-word answers eventually forced Dorothy to move on.

There was little else to do. Dorothy wandered about the empty building, standing alone in darkened rooms, trying to visualize the club before the war. In the dining room, she remembered sitting at a table for two, across from a smiling officer. In her mind, she saw the crisp tablecloth and the dapper waiter in his uniform. She pictured the twinkle of the tabletop candles and recalled the weight of the polished silverware in her hand.

She leaned against the doorframe and thought of the many times she was shown to her seat. She remembered taking a mental inventory as she crossed the dining room, seeing who was out for the evening

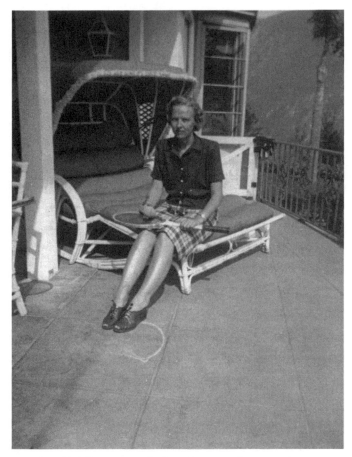

Dorothy off shift at Cavite before the war. The navy nurses worked half shifts due to the heat and had time for tennis, golf, and swimming. *Courtesy of Bureau of Medicine and Surgery*

and how the other ladies were dressed. There was one officer in particular who was her steady date. But they'd argued just before Pearl Harbor because she felt he wasn't serious about her. Now she had no idea whether he was still alive or what his future held. All she knew was that he was on the USS *Houston.*

Dorothy didn't know where she belonged. Many of the navy men who remained in the Philippines had transferred to the army to continue fighting the enemy. Dorothy wasn't sure what would happen to her and the other nurses, but she felt a flash of hope when the army began evacuating their medical corps. Dorothy and Susie said good-bye to the army surgeons headed to the field hospitals, and anticipated their own orders were coming soon.

On December 26, Susie and Dorothy received word that the navy nurses had their orders. Both women packed their belongings and then watched a corpsman heave their trunks into the back of a boxy station wagon. The women slid into the car, uncertain as to where they were headed. Would they set up a field hospital in Bataan? Or head to Corregidor, where the US military had a labyrinth of underground tunnels?

Processions of army vehicles sped north. As the corpsman put the car in gear and began driving, Dorothy expected him to slowly wedge the wagon into the heavy traffic. But he turned south and zoomed toward Santa Scholastica, a women's college that had been converted into a hospital.

"We're not going anywhere," the corpsman admitted.

Dorothy felt deflated. She watched from the windows as trucks carrying soldiers and supplies flowed from the capital. The road south was empty. No one wanted to be in Manila when the Japanese arrived. At Santa Scholastica, Dorothy climbed out of the wagon with concealed trepidation. What would happen to the navy nurses once the Japanese took hold? The Geneva Convention dictated that medical corps should not be made prisoners of war. But the Japanese had never ratified the convention. The nurses could only hope the Japanese would follow rules of engagement.

Hope dwindled during the next few days. Both the army and navy transferred their extremely ill and severely wounded patients to Santa Scholastica. It was clear to the nurses that these men would not be joining troops in Bataan or Corregidor. US commanders expected these patients to die before the enemy invaded the capital, or perhaps shortly thereafter. In the days leading up to the new year, the nurses developed a morbid routine of checking on patients to see if they were still alive. The wards felt like death's waiting room, and Dorothy and the other nurses wondered if they had received their own death sentences.

Part II

1942

4

Banzai

DOROTHY STOOD ON Santa Scholastica's rooftop, holding a glass of scotch on the rocks. It was almost midnight on New Year's Eve. A few of the medical staff bunched on the dark roof and admired the twinkling lights below. The roof gave them a fleeting gust of freedom. The former women's college felt like a holding pen. After MacArthur declared Manila an open city, scouts tore through the local hospitals to ensure every sailor or soldier was located and transferred to the makeshift hospital. Between December 27 and 30, ninety patients were admitted. Then, on December 31, the army briskly loaded its sixty-six patients onto a hospital ship. The holding pen suddenly felt like a cage, in which some occupants were released and others were trapped.

The navy's desertion was deliberate, and only one nurse was spared. Ann Bernatitus, who had lamented when she drew the short straw a few weeks back, quickly proved herself invaluable to an army surgeon. He insisted she evacuate to Bataan and assist him at Hospital No. 1. Both the army and navy approved the transfer. None of the navy nurses understood Ann's sudden departure. Several suspected she'd gone Absent Without Official Leave, or AWOL. Nurse Peg supported this theory and thought Ann deserved a court-martial. Ann's good friend, nurse Mary Chapman, was tearful over the loss of her friend. A few of the nurses pumped Dorothy for information after she disclosed how she was the last to see the missing nurse.

The brief encounter had happened on Christmas Eve when Dorothy wandered outside the Jai Alai Building, where fifty nurses waited to board buses for a field hospital in Bataan. It was early, just after 6:00 AM, and Ann sat on the curb, trying to stay out of the way. "What are you doing here?" Dorothy asked.

"I'm going to Bataan."

"Where's that?"

"I don't know," Ann admitted. "I just heard of it two days ago."

That was all Dorothy had to report. Chief Nurse Cobb had little else to share with her nurses, except that the fleet surgeon ordered the eleven remaining nurses to stay together until further notice. The women were hopeful during the following week that evacuation orders were indeed coming through. One of the captains even directed the women to keep their belongings packed, and Dorothy was optimistic the navy had a plan.

After the army evacuation, bitterness from the abandonment soured all hope. The Japanese were advancing, and it was only a matter of hours before Manila was occupied. In preparation, the navy men and women lowered the American flag and burned it to prevent the Japanese from disrespecting it. Several people blinked back tears of defeat as the flames licked the stripes.

By New Year's Eve, none of the medical personnel felt celebratory as the clock ticked toward midnight. Dorothy followed the others up to the school's roof. The air raids had stopped after Manila was declared an open city and the lights were back on. For a moment, the flickering lights gave the capital an illusion of normalcy, as if the Japanese were not expected to occupy the city within the next few days, as if most of the civilian population hadn't fled in fear. Dorothy raised her glass along with the others. They toasted each other. They toasted 1942, whatever it may bring.

The only orders the navy nurses received the next day were to stay within the confines of the college. From the windows, they watched as the Japanese wheeled into Manila on bicycles. The soldiers wore high, almost pointed helmets and supply bags with a cross-chest strap. They would have resembled newspaper delivery boys if it weren't for the menacing bayonets strapped across their backs. The Japanese soldiers did not bother with Santa Scholastica on their first day in the capital. But Dorothy and the others heard the nearby stadium erupt in cheers when the soldiers rolled up to the gate and released Japanese civilians from their internment.

"Banzai! Banzai!" the freed prisoners whooped.

Dorothy heard the excited battle cry from a block away. Everyone waited with anticipation, wondering when a Japanese commander would stride into the hospital and declare them all prisoners of the Empire of Japan. The naval captains were unsure what to expect from their captors, and they ordered all medical staff to receive cholera and dysentery vaccines.

A sense of powerlessness permeated as the staff rolled up their sleeves and lined up for vaccinations. There were 25 officers, 5 pharmacists, 102 corpsmen, and 161 patients (both Filipino and American). The 11 navy nurses were the only women, with the exception of Basilia Torres Steward, the Filipina wife of a naval officer.

Basilia was a small woman with thick, dark hair and puffy cheeks. She had a tendency when she was intently listening to lower her chin and turn her head to the side. At Santa Scholastica, she sat by her husband Jerry's bedside and tilted her head as he confided his fears.

Jerry had been stationed in the power plant at Cavite, and he was shot in the chest during the attack. He also had shrapnel wounds all over his body, including a painful one in his leg that was not healing well. Jerry, however, was more worried about his wife. He heard of the savagery of the Japanese army. Japanese soldiers had massacred Chinese citizens when they conquered the mainland. He knew Basilia's life was in Manila, but he wanted her to remain with the Americans. Basilia was a registered nurse, and Jerry planned to ask Chief Nurse Cobb to absorb her into her unit. Since they were noncombatants, Jerry expected the nurses to be repatriated. Jerry's family was in East Texas. Basilia, he hoped, could wait out the war with them.

Cobb had no objection, and she was pleased to have Basilia join her ranks. Basilia was an organized nurse who kept her own living space meticulous—a quality Cobb wished her young nurses would emulate. She had also been a chief nurse at a hospital in Manila, and she was clearly accomplished. The other nurses were also glad to include Basilia and commented how it seemed appropriate they were back to twelve. Quietly, Peg confided in Dorothy that she felt relieved the twelfth woman was Basilia and not missing nurse Ann Bernatitus. Peg and Ann never got along well, and Peg sensed she was about to be confined to close quarters with these women.

Basilia was fitted with a uniform to match the other nurses. As far as the Japanese Imperial Army was concerned, Basilia Torres Steward was a member of the Navy Nurse Corps. The invading army, however, would pay little attention to the navy nurses. In the coming years, the nurses learned the Japanese were never quite sure how to interpret the presence of female army or navy nurses. They did not view women as equal and never considered that the women might be military officers. In this sense, Jerry's protective instincts for his wife proved correct. As a passing member of the Navy Nurse Corps, Basilia was spared from the atrocities that later befell the citizens of Manila. And as a woman, the Japanese perceived her as a noncombatant and she was spared the agony her husband endured as a captured sailor. The guards weren't gentle with the women, but their deepest hatred was directed elsewhere.

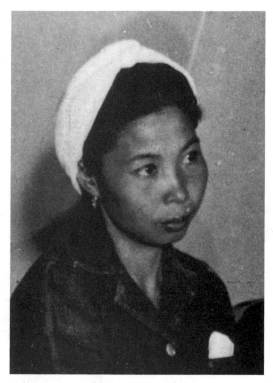

Civilian nurse Basilia Torres Steward. *Courtesy of Bureau of Medicine and Surgery*

Three Japanese soldiers stood at the front door. They paused a moment and then pounded their rifle butts against the wood. The hollow sound vibrated through the tense hallways. Captain Davis calmly opened the door and stood back as the soldiers pushed inside. Through an interpreter, the staff and patients were informed they were now prisoners of war.

The capture was calm, almost transactional. The Japanese announced the imprisonment, and the new captives accepted their fate stoically. Dorothy and the other nurses did not cry or panic. Per Captain Davis's instructions, the women continued nursing in the wards as though it were any other day. Several officers whispered assurances to the women that their detention was temporary. Soon they'd find themselves standing along Manila Bay, boarding a transport ship to Australia or the Indies. Such assurances, although well intended, were misinformed. In December, Guam had fallen to the Japanese after a few hours of resistance. The five US Navy nurses there had been afforded no special privileges. The women were confined to the naval hospital in Guam until the Japanese transferred them to a prisoner of war camp in Japan.

Captain Davis had ordered all medical personnel back into their white uniforms with the intention that the Japanese soldiers would leave the noncombatants unmolested. The three Japanese soldiers did not acknowledge the women on the first day. They checked the contents of the safe, posted several sentries out front, and left their captives to mind themselves. When the Japanese returned, they sent several California-educated naval officers who spoke fluent, gentlemanly English. They were courteous and chatted amiably with their American prisoners, explaining how they never wanted the war. But within a few days, the officers were replaced with aggressive guards from the Japanese army. The new guards looped barbed wire around the campus, sending a powerful message of defeat to those locked inside.

Within the coming days, the men were relieved of their sidearms and all ammunition was confiscated. The captives never planned a resistance, but the loss of the weapons was a defeating reminder they were defenseless and alone. Complete submission was the only option. The captives' compliance was first tested by their captors' pilfering. The guards greedily searched the men's belongings and cheerfully helped themselves to any item of interest. During head counts, Dorothy diverted her eyes as menacing sentries patted down corpsmen and officers. Watches, rings, and pens were all pocketed with a smug smile. Dorothy and the other nurses lost their utility knives and flashlights, but the Japanese did not bother searching the nurses' clothing trunks.

For a culture so obsessed with honor, the Japanese soldiers' thieving came as a surprise. To a certain extent, it stemmed from necessity. The Japanese military chose not to supply its troops with basic provisions. Soldiers were expected to be resourceful and fend for themselves. Fishing, gathering wild-growing fruits, or hunting meat helped troops in remote areas to cover the shortage. Occupying soldiers in urban settings had it much easier. They simply stole from civilians or prisoners.

In the quiet of the nurses' quarters, Dorothy watched as Peg opened a jar of cold cream. She pulled off her engagement ring and pushed it deep within the cream. The guards were unlikely to care about a woman's cosmetic, so it seemed a good hiding place. Peg looked at Dorothy as she tightened the lid and thought aloud as to why she hadn't married her fiancé, Edwin Wood, in Guam when she had the chance. The navy would have discharged her immediately and shipped her back to Pennsylvania.

Peg likely did not know that her fiancé was also a prisoner of war. Edwin was the executive officer on the USS *Penguin*, a minesweeper. The *Penguin* had darted out to sea when Japan attacked Guam. The antiaircraft battery was able to take down one of the enemy aircraft, but the satisfaction was short lived. The Japanese bombers persisted in waves, circling over the minesweeper and striving for a direct hit. Edwin raced down to the engineering room, ordering all the men onto lifeboats. The crew intentionally opened the sea valves and water rushed into the vessel. From his life raft, Edwin and the other men watched as the American flag atop the minesweeper slipped under the waterline.

Peg placed the cold cream jar with her other belongings. She wouldn't be needing the ring. Her February wedding was canceled, due to the bride being a prisoner of war. In his brief experience as a captive, Edwin was already well versed in the Japanese military's culture of violence. Peg and the other nurses would soon learn.

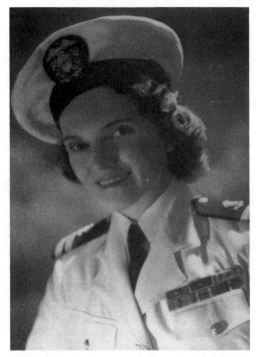

Navy nurse Margaret "Peg" Nash. *Courtesy of Women's Memorial Foundation Collection*

Chief Nurse Laura Cobb stood in front of a Japanese soldier, watching as he scrutinized the document in front of him. The soldier looked up at the medicine cabinet and pulled out one of the bottles to examine the label. He replaced the bottle on the shelf and moved to the next item on the list. He was there to raid the pharmaceutical supply and had orders to bring back any valuable drugs, especially quinine to treat malaria. The mosquito-borne disease caused high fevers, vomiting, and exhaustion. Symptoms took as long as two weeks to emerge, and the most severe patients were at risk of slipping into a seizure or coma. Back at Cavite, the nurses typically mixed the quinine powder with water and had the patient drink the formula several times a day. The doses decreased as the patient improved, which was the expected outcome.

Earlier, the Japanese guards had ordered Cobb to create an inventory list of all drugs, and she'd strategized on how to keep the key pharmaceuticals. Cobb worried that the medical corps would soon become patients themselves. The quinine had to remain in her possession. Who knew how deep into the jungles the captors intended to send her nurses?

Shorting the inventory list was not a safe option. The Japanese were beginning to conduct exhaustive searches on a daily basis, and they would likely find the hidden medicines that Cobb claimed did not exist. A falsified inventory list could serve as her death warrant if an angry guard decided her dishonesty deserved summary execution.

Cobb considered other options. The guards had yet to bother with the women's personal items, and it was possible for each nurse to tuck a vial of morphine or a bottle of quinine into her trunk. But what would happen if the guards ransacked the women's belongings and found medicines rolled into sanitary napkins or stockings? Cobb could not risk retribution against her nurses. Another possibility was for each nurse to conceal a bottle on her body. It was a successful tactic for their army counterparts. Before they left Manila, the army nurses were instructed to tuck a vial of morphine into their hair. The women were advised to save the morphine until desperation demanded their last dose. But tucking medicine vials under caps wasn't enough. Cobb didn't know how long she and her nurses would be detained. Most of the nurses anticipated it would take several months for the Allied forces to push the Japanese out of the Philippines. Until then, Cobb needed more medicine than Dorothy's blond curls or Mary Rose's auburn tresses could conceal.

The solution soon presented itself. The Japanese guards plundered only items they perceived as valuable. Cobb simply needed to make her medicines less desirable. She ordered her nurses to switch the quinine in the bottles with sodium bicarbonate, also known as baking soda.

The soldier examining the medicine cabinet seemed primarily focused on confirming that the inventory was fully disclosed. With that task complete, he moved on to the next order of business—removing the entire quinine supply. It did not occur to him that he should dab a sample on his tongue to verify the powder had the drug's distinct bitter taste. Instead, he hastily loaded up the bottles and ferried them from the school, seemingly certain the Japanese medical corps would be delighted to have such an ample stash.

Cobb likely smiled to herself as she closed the medicine cabinet and turned the key. The powder the soldier stole would not cure any case of malaria. It would be useful, however, for disinfecting their kitchen counters. Or should the Japanese medical corps desire to bake a cake that called for an acidic ingredient such as lemon, then they would have the baking soda needed to make the batter rise.

5

Chin Up, Girls

———————

NURSE EDWINA TODD woke suddenly. She did not have her glasses on, but she sensed danger. In the dark, a Japanese sentry hovered over her bed. Her mosquito net was slightly raised, and the soldier had slid his bayonet under the mesh. The knife tip was inches away from her body. The guard was apparently waiting for Edwina to sense his presence and wake up.

When the guard saw Edwina was awake, he held the knife point steady. Her blood quickened as she stiffened with fear. She'd have no choice but to comply if he ordered her out of bed. She was at his mercy. The sentry allowed the suspense to build. Would he force her from bed at knifepoint and violate her in another room? Or did he intend to kill her? Edwina blinked at the fuzzy form who wielded absolute control over her. She watched anxiously as he withdrew his knife and walked away.

Edwina lay in bed, waiting for the rush of adrenaline to dissolve. Sleep seemed pointless. As soon as she drifted off, another guard would stride to the middle of the room and stomp his feet. The sentries barged through the room periodically at night and then took pleasure in watching the fatigued nurses move sluggishly the next day.

Cobb was powerless to stop the harassment, but she tried to protect her nurses. She implemented a curfew so that all nurses were within the safety of the pack by 9:00 PM. Most of the patients who were gravely ill or injured had died, and the corpsmen were capable of managing the remaining patients during the overnight hours. And not all the men needed their help. The patient census now included fully recovered men who intentionally remained in bed in hopes of avoiding forced labor. The guards, however, accepted no excuses as to why a man was unable to participate, and about forty men were drafted each day. Dorothy watched with sorrow as men with broken bones or infectious diseases were ordered to join a work detail. The men staggered from bed and limped down the ward and into the tropical sun for a day of slave labor. The more able-bodied tried to help the infirmed with their loads, but Dorothy knew that merely being out of bed was agonizing.

Dorothy increasingly felt her fellow prisoners' pain. She stung with humiliation after a guard violently slapped a gentle physician across the face. The physician had tried to comfort two young sentries who startled after bombs exploded at a nearby airfield. The guards panicked at the thundering boom, and the doctor encouraged them to step inside the building. Rather than appreciating the kindness, one of the guards was insulted by what he perceived as a patronizing gesture.

The prisoners referred to the pummeling as "slaps," but the force was far more severe. The close-range blows knocked teeth loose and broke jaws. Few men escaped the guards' punishments, and there were naval officers who had to visit oral surgeons after the war to repair loose molars. Even patients who were too ill to bow to the guards were slapped in retribution. The physical punishments were subjective and hard to predict. The prisoners soon learned that what one guard tolerated, another punished.

The Japanese armed forces allowed for such violence as part of their culture of obedience and honor. Within the Japanese military, anyone of a higher rank had the authority to slap or physically punish anyone of a lower rank. The guards who lorded over the camps were mostly low-ranking members of the military who had endured their own history of slaps. The prisoners were natural targets for their newly acquired power.

The nurses were surprised to see how the Japanese disciplined their own. On one occasion, a few bored corpsmen strung a volleyball net across the courtyard and began a game. Several young guards accepted the corpsmen's offer to join the game. The sentries left their bayonets on the ground and took their place on the makeshift court. When the sergeant strode into the courtyard, he saw his unarmed soldiers happily volleying the ball. The yard went silent as the sergeant berated the guards and cracked them across the face. Dietitian Bertha felt sympathy and winced as the young guards were hit. At thirty-seven, she was almost two decades older. She saw them as homesick boys who never asked for war.

It was one of the few times the nurses felt sorry for their captors, especially as life became increasingly difficult. The officers in charge were progressively sadistic. At the end of January, they ordered the removal of all patient bed frames, mattresses, linens, pajamas, and mosquito nets. Thirty patients were whisked away to an elementary school that was halfheartedly converted into a prison/hospital. The officers assured the medical corps the new hospital was well equipped, but Dorothy later heard that patients there were sleeping on the ground and drinking from a dirty, dribbling tap.

Then in mid-February, the prison population at Santa Scholastica dropped dramatically. The guards ordered their captives to complete forms listing their name, age, birthplace, next of kin, education, religion, and naval rank. The forms were given to Captain Davis, who was directed to select ninety-two men for transfer by the end of the week. No one knew where the men were being sent. The commander assured Captain Davis the men were being transferred to a "well-equipped" hospital. But the prisoners worried they were headed for a mass grave. The Japanese were operating with their own rule book, one in which surrender did not guarantee safety.

February 14 was a clear morning near the Dutch Indies. The waves were calm and the sun was shining. Australian Army nurse Vivian Bullwinkel stood on the deck of an evacuation vessel and relished the tranquility. The past few months had been as stressful for the Australian nurses as for their American counterparts in the Philippines.

Vivian had been posted in Singapore when the Japanese attacked Pearl Harbor and then turned their attention to British Malaya. British forces resisted for two months. But by mid-February, almost sixty thousand British troops were defeated and forced to surrender. Severely injured men, their nurses, and stranded civilians were loaded onto evacuation ships in advance of the enemy occupation. At the wharf, Vivian passed lines of anxious civilians trying to find passage from the fallen city. The bay was littered with the masts of sunken ships.

Many of the nurses were upset about leaving their patients and glumly boarded the dark gray evacuation yacht. Others were eager to escape the imminent occupation and felt relieved as the boat left the smoldering city. The overnight hours, however, brought new perils. The yacht was part of a convoy that came close to a naval battle. The unnerved captain lost contact with the convoy and was now navigating his ship through mine-infested waters. Vivian and the other nurses were unaware the yacht was alone and anchored in a minefield. To Vivian, the morning seemed perfectly placid, and she drank in the view of a sandy beach.

The calm was broken without warning. A formation of Japanese planes flew low, propelling toward the yacht with machine guns firing at the upper deck. Vivian felt the ship's urgent motion as the captain up-anchored and fled for open waters. The next few hours were filled with nervous chatter as the passengers realized the Japanese were gunning for them.

It did not take long for the Japanese military to resume its attack. Around two o'clock, a new formation sped toward the yacht and released three bombs. A shrieking whistle blew in response, directing all the passengers to abandon the ship and climb into lifeboats. Vivian and the other nurses helped the elderly and infirmed into rafts. The lifeboats quickly filled to capacity, leaving dozens of nurses stranded on the deck. The remaining nurses were ordered to kick off their shoes, jump in the water, and swim away from the sinking yacht.

Vivian was able to find a spot in a raft, and the evacuees pushed themselves from the doomed vessel. They floated under the gauze of dark smoke blocking the sun. The water beneath their boat turned inky as the oil from the sunken ship erupted on the surface. Vivian called to the nurses in the water, but the women were slick with oil and unable to grip the rafts. The waves pulled them away.

Vivian and twenty-one of her fellow nurses washed up near Radjik Beach on the small island of Bangka. The survivors pulled the rafts onto the shore and staggered onto the sand. There were about one hundred wet and shaken people huddled on the beach. The group remained for two days, hoping a rescue boat might ferry them to Australia. They learned from the locals that the small island was under enemy control. Eventually one of the yacht's officers resolved to surrender and set off to find a Japanese commander.

Matron Irene Melville Drummond ordered her nurses to remain with their patients. She expected that the shelter they built with a large red cross would properly signify they were medical corps. But she also sensed the unpredictability of the situation. She recommended that the civilian women and children on the beach promptly leave and walk toward the nearest town. After the civilians departed, the yacht officer returned with twenty Japanese soldiers and one commander.

The men were separated from the twenty-two nurses. Ambulatory men were ordered to march, and the nurses watched them until they slipped beyond a small bluff. The women heard the staccato of machine gun fire. Screams of men being sliced with bayonets ripped through the sounds of the surf. The nurses looked at each other in alarm. "They are not taking prisoners!" they repeated in a panic.

The Japanese returned to the beach, eyeing the nurses and their incapacitated patients. The soldiers made a sadistic show of slowly wiping the blood from their bayonet tips. Several soldiers began setting up a machine gun. They pointed the gun at the waves and ordered the women into the surf. The nurses clutched each other and waded into the water.

Matron Drummond knew the soldiers intended to murder them all. "Chin up, girls," she called. "I'm proud of you and I love you all."

The women collapsed into the waves. A few of the women were killed on impact. Others were incapacitated and drowned. Vivian felt a searing pain in her side. She was hit by a single bullet that missed every major organ and artery. She closed her eyes and floated on her back, pretending to be dead as the Japanese sliced and stabbed the patients on the beach.

The bodies of her friends were battered back and forth in the waves. Vivian pushed herself to keep a safe distance. She bobbed for hours in the salt water, forcing herself to appear lifeless. When she sensed the soldiers had departed, she treaded water and surveyed the maimed corpses on the blood-saturated sand. Vivian swam toward the shore and stepped through the carnage. She was the only woman to survive the massacre. Among the dead, she found one injured soldier who had also lived through the ordeal. She cared for him for weeks in the jungle wilds until the locals indicated that their willingness to help was nearly exhausted. Vivian and her injured soldier wandered along a road until a passing car with Japanese officers pulled up and promptly arrested them.

The officers brought Vivian to a local jail where other nurses who'd survived the sinking of the yacht were being held captive. Most of them were still shoeless and had uncomfortable chin gashes from where their life vests had rubbed off the skin. Vivian whispered the story of the slaughter to the other nurses. They vowed not to speak of it for the rest of their imprisonment. They feared their captors' response if they found a survivor. They pledged upon their release to tell Australia and the world that the Japanese treated women, children, medical corps, and noncombatants as enemies. There was no mercy, not even for nurses.

Chief Nurse Laura Cobb appeared calm on the surface. Dorothy thought she looked like her usual ill-humored self. Cobb was tense, and there was a sharpness to her voice that suggested none of the nurses should test her. The women did not know the true cause of her foul mood. Cobb was insulating them from the terrifying prospect that one of them was hours away from execution.

An American fleet reservist had escaped. Nurse Peg Nash was on duty in the ward the morning after the escape and lined up with her patients for the morning head count. The prisoners bowed to the sentry and then heard him count down the line in Japanese: *ichi, ni, san.* Several of the patients stood nervously, waiting for the guard to discover what they already knew. The guard reached the end of the line and turned back, quietly counting to himself.

Peg assumed the situation was no longer her problem. But the guard wanted immediate retribution and demanded the summary execution of Captain Davis, as well as the corpsmen and nurse on duty in the ward. "Shoot nurses too!" he insisted.

The sentry reported the escape to his superior, who contacted the Japanese military police in order to launch a full investigation. The military police outranked the guard and ordered him to suspend the executions while they completed their work. The prisoners whispered broken bits of information in the interim, warning each other of the promised terror. In the ward, Peg knew Captain Davis and the corpsmen were marked for execution. She did not realize she was included in the lineup as well.

Cobb soon saw the small, dark-haired nurse hurrying over with a concerned look on her face. Peg confided that she was fearful one of her corpsmen was going to be killed. Cobb studied the young woman and realized she still didn't know she herself had also been selected for execution. Cobb pressed her lips together and remained silent. She was not going to give Peg, or any of the other nurses, reason to worry. But she had every reason to fear they would be burying Peg before sundown.

Peg had the habit of smiling, even when something pained her. It was a nervous type of smile that slowed her speech as she carefully enunciated her words. Her constant smile was intended to make others around her more comfortable. But it likely pained Cobb to see the condemned woman unwittingly trying to make the situation easier for others. Tension strangled the small prison as the morning progressed. Dorothy and the other nurses reacted to sudden movements or loud sounds. No one was certain how the execution would proceed, but it was anticipated the guards would order the entire prison to line up and witness the brutality.

Within a few hours, Dorothy saw notices posted around the building. She approached one of the neatly printed pages and saw it was a warning. If anyone else escaped, the two men who slept on each side of the escapee would be executed, along with the nurse on duty. The note was a reprieve for the prisoners already slated for death.

The military police apparently did not care to spend time on the issue. Especially when the Japanese army had other plans.

———————

Cobb withheld news of another crisis from her nurses. She kept the concern to herself and lay in bed worrying about their fate. It was impossible to predict what might happen to them. In the two months they'd been held captive, all her expectations were shattered and then replaced with new assumptions that never came to fruition. Now she had troubling new information she hoped would prove false. The Japanese army, she'd learned, intended to transfer half of the nurses to a civilian prison camp. Cobb sensed such a transfer meant indefinite incarceration. All hope of repatriation would be gone.

Cobb received her information from Captain Davis, who was doing a poor job of negotiating on behalf of Cobb and her nurses. Davis knew the Japanese army was liquidating the hospital and transferring patients to the makeshift prison at the elementary school. Davis likely thought he was securing a safe place for the nurses, but Cobb was horrified by his suggestions. She quickly rejected his idea of separating the women. Problematically, Davis had already spoken with his Japanese counterpart and the separation seemed likely. Cobb was tormented by the prospect. How could she choose who stayed and who left? What if the women were abused in the civilian camp? Cobb plotted the possibilities in her head. She knew their incarceration would last until the Allies regained control of the islands, which she now expected might not be for many months.

In the darkness, Dorothy disrupted Cobb's thoughts. The young nurse was clearly uncomfortable. She shifted positions and then kicked off her sheet. A moment later, she covered herself as though she had the chills. She rose suddenly, the sound of her bare feet smacking down the dormitory toward the bathroom. Cobb promptly followed.

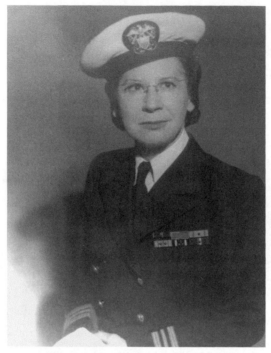

Chief Nurse Laura Cobb. *Courtesy of Bureau of Medicine and Surgery*

Dorothy retched into the toilet. Cobb heard her gag, breathe, and then flush. Dorothy emerged from the bathroom stall, sick and shaken. Cobb looked at the young woman's yellow eyes and immediately knew she had infectious hepatitis. Dorothy had picked up the disease either through a food-borne illness or by coming into contact with contaminated blood or fecal matter. The latter was most likely. The guards had restricted the laundry facilities, which meant the nurses now helped the corpsmen keep up with the laundry. A few weeks back, Dorothy hung wet laundry on lines in the courtyard. Soap alone could not rinse out hepatitis A, and Dorothy likely contracted the virus as she pinned linens to the line.

Cobb was fearful for Dorothy, but her terse response made her seem irritated. "I'm sorry?" Dorothy apologized.

"You're not as sorry as I am," Cobb shot back.

Dorothy sulkily followed her superior back into the dormitory. She was flush with fever and angry with her superior. It wasn't her fault, she thought, that she had hepatitis. She didn't *choose* to be infected. Cobb ordered Dorothy to bed and limited her to a liquid diet.

Dorothy primarily slept the next few days, occasionally awakened by the nurses' conversations. Cobb's stress was contagious and spread among her subordinates. The women understood something was amiss, but they didn't fully understand the threat, which only served to heighten their anxieties.

Cobb's new source of stress, however, was personal. Captain Davis had returned to the Japanese commander at Cobb's urging and asked if the women could stay together. The commander agreed the nurses could remain intact as a unit—but without their leader. Cobb would be required to stay behind at the college with the men. Cobb concealed her anxiousness with irritation. Her bad mood was convincing to nurses like Dorothy who assumed Cobb was just being her typical, sourpuss self. Cobb's closer friends sensed her underlying tension and began to act out their anxieties. The corpsmen gossiped specifically about Edwina, who they alleged was not proving as resilient. There were rumors that her behavior had been erratic and emotional.

Edwina had always been a woman with her own quirks. She lacked coordination, and Dorothy had spent many afternoons on the golf course watching Edwina swing and miss. She was sharp and lively during her shifts but scattered in her personal life. In their time at Cavite, Dorothy had often waited in the hallway of the nurses' quarters while Edwina searched for a missing shoe. Dorothy was well accustomed to Edwina's oddities, which over the years she'd found increasingly charming. The corpsmen didn't know Edwina as well. They only saw a nurse slamming doors, barking orders, and tearing up in front of patients.

Dietitian Bertha Evans updated Dorothy about the Edwina rumors. Bertha had come to check on Dorothy and see if she was ready to stomach a soft diet. She brought Dorothy up to date on the gossip she had missed during her illness. There were whispers that several of the corpsmen had reported Edwina's conduct to Captain Davis. Bertha confided that Edwina was not the same person she had been a few weeks before, and it seemed hard to talk with her. It was true, Dorothy acknowledged, that Edwina had been a bit unhinged, but she didn't think her conduct warranted a report to the captain.

Dorothy fell asleep after Bertha left. She was awakened abruptly by the clicking heels of an angry woman, striding in her direction. Edwina understood people were talking about her, and she was furious about the gossip. Dorothy was the weakest person in the nurses' quarters and she seemed a suitable target for Edwina's hurt feelings.

Dorothy opened her eyes and saw Edwina's face. Edwina shook her finger and hissed a warning. If Dorothy had anything to say about her, then she'd better say it to her face! She stomped out of the quarters, leaving Dorothy stunned in her bed. Dorothy expected viciousness from her captors, not her fellow inmates. The indignities of incarceration seemed to find new ways to breed.

Dorothy was still not well when the commander ordered the women to the courtyard. Cobb sensed a pending announcement and steeled herself to appear composed. The women waited quietly for the interpreter. He briskly interpreted the message—the women were to be transferred that afternoon to Santo Tomas prison camp.

"Are we all to go?" Cobb asked hopefully.

"Yes," the interpreter confirmed.

The women were directed to pack all their belongings. They were allowed to bring their mattresses, as those were a gift from the

Japanese naval officers. Their trunks were permitted as well, along with basic cookware, dinnerware, and laundry supplies.

Corpsmen helped Dorothy carry her belongings to the staging area and tried to be optimistic. One corpsman said the nurses were headed to a better place. A few relied on humor to ease the separation and joked how they'd keep the other corpsmen in line. Dorothy smiled weakly at the men pushing her trunk into the courtyard. She did not know where they were headed and if they would ever see each other again.

Captain Davis came to wish the women well and then delivered a sober warning. The civilian camps were plagued with informants. Most of these amateur spies were other prisoners who traded information for privileges. As military women, the nurses would be ideal targets. An informant might try to build a nurse's trust in order to collect information about the US Navy. Be courteous, he advised, but do not make friends with the civilians.

Cobb stood amid the group, listening to the captain's advice. She intended to keep her eleven nurses together. She planned to order the women to maintain their status as navy nurses. Surely the civilian camp had an infirmary that required their services. If so, Cobb would assign her nurses daily shifts and provide medical services until their liberation. None of the women had joined the navy to treat civilians, but Cobb trusted her nurses would accept their new role without complaint.

Dorothy glanced over at Cobb and thought she looked ridiculous. Her chief nurse wore a type of lei around her neck as if they were attending an island theme party at an officers' club. Dorothy was quietly annoyed. They were headed to a *prison* camp—there was no cause for celebration. Another nurse noticed Dorothy's irritated expression. The lei, the nurse explained, was a cover-up. Cobb had tucked the nurses' military records underneath her uniform. The documents formed an incriminating square across her chest, which Cobb concealed with the string of flowers.

Preserving the records meant the navy could never question or deny the nurses' service. Cobb ensured her nurses would be recognized for their continued service and eligible for every increase in salary. Private records were forbidden in Japanese POW camps, and the women felt uneasy in knowing their chief nurse was willing to go to this extreme. It seemed ominous, as though Cobb suspected something they did not. Secret records in a prison camp weren't just an act of resistance—they created a paper trail that could stand as witness to atrocities if the victims were one day unable to speak for themselves.

The women bit back their emotions as they said good-bye to the other medical personnel. The sense of isolation as they separated from their countrymen was defeating. There were 102 corpsmen at the makeshift prison, and almost half had been with the nurses since their time at Cavite. The men who loaded the nurses' luggage into the car trunks and hugged them good-bye were the same ones they'd relied on during those brutal, bloody hours after the bombing. The nurses had bonded with their corpsmen in the three months since the attack. Together they experienced the alternating waves of terror and boredom that delineated the war. And they collectively felt the humiliation, pain, and fear that defined their POW experience.

The twelve women were divided and ordered into the cars. The nurses and the corpsmen exchanged comforting smiles and small waves, silently wishing the best for each other. As the car doors slammed, the nurses left men who were destined for agony. The corpsmen at Santa Scholastica would suffer exponentially in the coming months. Most did not survive the war. Of the 102 corpsmen, only 30 lived through the ordeal.

Most of the corpsmen would survive until the end of 1944. At that time, the Allied forces were gaining ground in the Pacific and the Allies were mere weeks from reclaiming the Philippines. The Japanese army did not want to face the embarrassment of their captives celebrating their capitulation. They began transporting thousands of prisoners to forced labor camps in Japan.

The prisoners called them "hell ships," and fifty-four of Dorothy's corpsmen were drafted onto the *Arisan Maru* in October 1944. The once-strapping corpsmen resembled skeletons as they lined up at the Manila dock and waited their turn to be stuffed into suffocating cargo holds. In the below-deck hold were wooden bunks stacked vertically. There was little room to move, and severely ill men were unable to push their way to the oversized canisters used as latrines. Men suffering from debilitating tropical diseases soiled themselves while whimpering apologies to the unfortunate prisoners trapped in the bunks below.

In their final days, the corpsmen blinked away the trickles of urine and splatters of diarrhea that streamed from above. Their emaciated frames displayed all the bones in their rib cages, and their joints pressed painfully on the wooden bunks. The hell ship guards showed no mercy. The corpsmen cried for water in scorching holds that burned at 120 degrees Fahrenheit. The men—the same ones who had chatted with Dorothy at Cavite, played rummy with her at the Jai Alai Building, and quietly performed impressions of the sentries at Santa Scholastica—were trapped for weeks on the miserable transports. Many lost their will to live, and openly wished for an American torpedo to end their misery. They did not have to wait long.

The Japanese ignored the international agreement that POW ships should be clearly marked, so the commanders of the US submarine hunting Japanese vessels in the South China Sea did not realize almost eighteen hundred POWs were aboard the *Arisan Maru*. In the confines of the holds, the trapped men heard the pings from the submarine's sonar bouncing off the vessel. Father John Scecina, an army chaplain from Indiana, began reciting the absolution: ". . . *augmentum gratiae et praemium vitae aeternae.*"

The prisoners felt the quake of the torpedo piercing the ship. They heard scurried footfalls as the Japanese crew scrambled into lifeboats. Within the hour, the prisoners realized the Japanese had abandoned the ship and they were free to hoist themselves from the holds. On the deck, the men saw only water surrounding them. The nearest island was 250 miles away.

Men with the will to live tried to swim or piece together rafts, but others thought it best to wait. They wanted to ride the suction of the sinking ship to the bottom of the ocean to ensure a faster death. Others stormed the canteen before the ocean could take them under and slurped handfuls of sugar. Many tried to find peace and sought a confession with Father Scecina.

Dozens of prisoners circled around Father Scecina as water filled the deck. There was no suction as the ship went under and the men suddenly found themselves in the cold water. Only eight of the eighteen hundred men survived. All of the fifty-four corpsmen from Santa Scholastica were killed. Two months later, twelve more of the corpsmen died when their hell ship, the *Ōryoku Maru*, was bombed by an American aircraft.

As the cars turned out of the campus drive two years earlier, the nurses and the corpsmen mercifully did not know what lay in wait.

6

Room 30A

––––––––––

DOROTHY LOOKED OUT the car window. She had not left Santa Scholastica since the occupation, and she sensed the four-mile drive would be one of her last glimpses of the outside world in the turbulent months to come. But what she saw depressed her. Manila was not the vibrant, cheerful city she recalled. The streets were void of locals, and the ominous passing of bicycling soldiers explained why the people of Manila were reluctant to venture out.

The city felt apocalyptic. Structures were bombed or burned into rubble. A shell of Manila remained, and its new occupants made it unrecognizable. The Japanese flag flew above seized buildings and soldiers clutching bayonets lorded in front of entryways. Dorothy felt disgusted when she saw large American automobiles chauffeuring Japanese officers. She was well aware of the confiscations but seeing the stolen cars in action deepened the insult.

The convoy soon stopped outside the curved gate of Santo Tomas. Dorothy saw hundreds of people crowding around the iron bars. Most were Filipino locals clutching packages they hoped to pass to a friend, former employer, or neighbor. The guards insisted on inspecting each package for covert communication. If a note was found, the package was destroyed and the deliverer received a sharp crack to the jawbone. Dorothy soon learned that for many prisoners those packages meant survival, and there would be no one on the other side of the gate for her.

The Japanese called the camp "protective custody," and believed this status absolved them of supplying the three thousand inmates at Santo Tomas with food, bedding, cooking supplies, soap, or even toilet paper. Few inmates were able to bring these necessities into the camp. Most showed up with only a suitcase after the invading army claimed the internment would last less than a week. Wealthy Americans, British, or Dutch were able to rely on friends, former neighbors, or faithful employees to pass supplies through the gate. The rest of the inmates scavenged.

Californian Margaret Sherk was one of the have-nots. She received pies a few times from a former neighbor and was delighted with them, particularly the secret notes tucked under the crust that wished her well and momentarily raised her spirits. But she burned with anger as other inmates boiled water in anticipation of dropping in rice or noodles. And she felt deprived whenever a prisoner peeled back the lid of a sardine can or biscuit tin. She had none of that for herself or David, her three-year-old son.

Margaret was twenty-six years old and the wife of a young mining engineer employed in the Philippines. They were civilians, and she'd watched with alarm when the army began sending dependents home during the summer of 1941. She considered returning to California, but an army official assured her the Philippines was the safest place in the Pacific. After Pearl Harbor, her husband, Bob, joined the army, which eagerly accepted him on the spot. Within weeks, she and David were ordered to report to Santo Tomas. She arrived with only a few suitcases. Now Margaret felt lied to, abandoned, and desperate. Like all the other inmates, she was assigned to a classroom that had been converted into a dormitory. Each inmate was allotted a mere twenty-two feet of living space. Margaret pushed her suitcases under her bed and tried to stash other supplies in her limited space whenever they became available.

Collecting necessities was a challenge, and Margaret resented the inmates who seemed to have everything. The most well-off built thatched shanties in the open-air courtyards of the main building. During the day they escaped to these little houses, where they cooked, read, and enjoyed having a barrier between themselves and other inmates. Meanwhile, Margaret and David stood three times a day in a slow-moving line at the prison's "restaurant," where their punch cards entitled them to a meager meal of rice, sweet potatoes, duck eggs (on a good day), or maybe a sardine. The lengthy line took an hour each time, and Margaret spent most of her day on her feet, waiting to eat or sip from the water fountain. The bathrooms involved the lengthiest wait. In the main building, six bathrooms serviced twenty-one hundred people—an average of a hundred inmates per toilet.

Parents with multiple children learned which one of their kids could be trusted to hold a place in line. The prison had a "canteen" where 250 products were sold at inflated prices. Some young internees were trusted by their parents to take a small stool and a picture book and wait quietly in the canteen line. But if a child wandered off to follow a stray kitty or a developing game of marbles, the parent might return after an hour to find that the family no longer had a place in the line and had to start over.

It was a problem that Margaret envied. She begrudged those with money for canteen purchases. And in the coming years, she would come to dislike the hundreds of inmates who received vendor licenses and lined the hallways with small displays of bakery goods, candies, and other items she could not secure for her hungry boy. Her anger depleted her sympathy for her fellow prisoners. In her mind, she formulated a

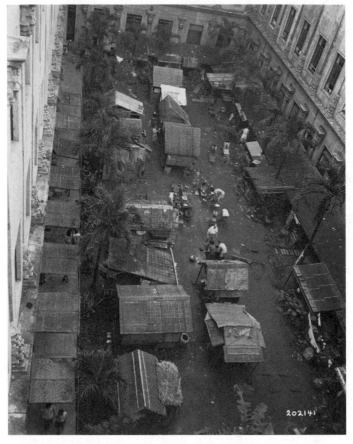

Inmates with financial means at Santo Tomas erected shanties in the courtyards where they could cook, eat, and find privacy amid the overcrowding. *Courtesy of National Archives, https://catalog.archives.gov/id/840222*

hierarchy of suffering. Her torment, she decided, was more severe than a woman who was raped. She rationalized that a woman who was raped only endured the trauma once, whereas she starved for years and was thus worthy of more compassion. She could not bring herself to care what others had seen or that their lives had been permanently altered.

Such was the environment the navy nurses were entering. They knew the guards would be hostile, but they likely did not realize there were inmates who were antagonistic and fought each other over perceived slights. Others, like Margaret, were overburdened and indifferent to others' sufferings. It was an odd invisibility. The prisoners were piled on top of each other, yet there were times they did not see each other at all.

Dorothy stood by the cars with the other nurses. The vehicles were a novelty, and a crowd of curious inmates gathered to see who had arrived. Dorothy looked at the camp and immediately determined that the former university had deteriorated into a slum. The main building was a massive square structure with two open-air courtyards in the middle. The front windows were covered with ratted, lice-infested blankets. Flies buzzed through the camp and mice slunk in the shadows.

The corpsmen at Santa Scholastica had optimistically insisted that the nurses were headed to a better place. Santo Tomas was worse. It was infested, overcrowded, and diseased. Dorothy was condemned to this hell. She retreated to the shade while Cobb went inside the building to meet with the inmates' elected leaders. The camp had an "executive committee" composed of inmates who were voted into office every few months. There were layers of subcommittees, hallway monitors, and room monitors who reported up to the executive committee. In the coming years, the executive committee proved protective of inmate interests. But it did not have the power to stop punishment, execution, or years of starvation.

Dorothy was summoned to rejoin the group. Before the women could settle in, they first had to stand for a group photograph. The camp commander, Ryozo Tsurumi, noticed that the nurses were slender but not emaciated, and they looked clean and well kempt in their uniforms. A photo of them would help him keep up appearances. Tsurumi was a civilian with the Japanese Consular Service. In comparison to other commandants, Tsurumi was fairly benign; he allowed the executive committee to manage daily life. Tsurumi's primary goal was to demonstrate to the Japanese Imperial Army that their faith in him was well deserved and the camp was in good order.

When the photo was taken, nurses Mary Chapman and Basilia Torres Steward had stepped away, but the guard photographing them didn't care about accuracy. It was for propaganda purposes, intended to suggest to the Red Cross and other meddling organizations that the inmates were treated well and in good health. The sentry stood with his back to the sun, and the nurses squinted in the light. Nurse anesthetist Susie Pitcher stood at the end, her cigarettes stuffed into her front pocket and her blond hair pulled back and fluffed, as if she'd hidden something in it. Helen Gorzelanski stood next to her and looked at the guard as though he was stupid. Peg Nash held her hands behind her back and furrowed her brow. Alongside her, Eldene Paige tilted her dark head. Chief Nurse Cobb stood to her right, a half step in front of her nurses, with her shoulders pulled back and an authoritative look on her face. Behind her, enigmatic Edwina Todd mustered a smile.

The taller women stood in the back row. The auburn-haired Mary Rose Harrington looked as though she was biting back tears. Next to her, surgical nurse Goldia O'Haver managed a smile. Dietitian Bertha Evans lowered her chin. Dorothy, on the end, was the only woman out of uniform. She wore a light-colored, belted dress, the type she would have worn on the voyage to the Philippines. Her hair was pulled back and she tucked her arms behind her back. Her lips pursed together, but she did not frown. Her tense eyes, however, revealed all her emotions. Dorothy was petrified.

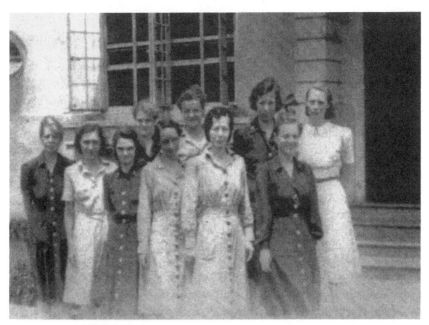

Upon arrival at Santo Tomas, the navy nurses were forced to pose for a Japanese propaganda photo. *Front row, left to right:* Susie Pitcher, Helen Gorzelanski, Peg Nash, Eldene Paige, Laura Cobb, Edwina Todd. *Back row, left to right:* Mary Rose Harrington, Goldia O'Haver, Bertha Evans, Dorothy Still. *Not pictured:* Mary Chapman and Basilia Torres Steward. *Courtesy of Bureau of Medicine and Surgery*

The nurses trudged up to room 30A, a former classroom now set aside to house women and older girls. The nurses were the first ones to occupy the room, and they promptly chose a corner space at the far end. It was the best real estate the former classroom had to offer. In comparison, Margaret Sherk and her son had spots by the door of their dormitory, which meant a constant parade of passersby. Dorothy and the other nurses set up their cots, slid their luggage underneath, and positioned their trunks as footlockers.

Across the hall, Dorothy glimpsed another dormitory and foresaw how 30A would look when it filled to capacity. All the dormitories had a narrow aisle which was meant to be kept open at all times. Slim cots lined each side of the aisle, carefully positioned to adhere to the twenty-two-square-feet limit. Mosquito nets draped across the room in large sheets and confined the space further. The inmates used every available inch to store cookware, clothing, eating utensils, cleaning instruments, and other daily necessities.

The room reached capacity the next day and 30A became a world unto itself. There were women from all over the globe of varying means, from modest missionaries to wives of wealthy executives. Some women were married to military men, others were prostitutes who came to the Philippines to take lonely servicemen's money. Dorothy was fascinated by a pair of Russian prostitutes, one of whom clearly had suffered scurvy as a child and walked on bowed legs. The women always dressed up in heels and slinky dresses, and they kept their space orderly. Dorothy had to admit such organization was not what she expected from two women who sold their bodies for a living.

Dorothy struggled to adjust to the new space and its inhabitants. The high ceilings meant that noise rolled constantly around the room. At night, she found it difficult to fall asleep among the constant inter-ruptions of creaking beds and snoring women. Her eyes closed only to suddenly open from the release of a horn-sounding sneeze. Once awake, she found herself focusing on Susie's wheezing exhales. The nurse anesthetist was only forty, but years of smoking labored her breathing. She was a beautiful woman with bright blond hair, full lips, and soft facial features that made her seem approachable. On the inside, her heart was damaged, and her lungs were black. Susie was not long for the world, and the stress of imprisonment fueled her nicotine addiction.

After midnight, the large windows in the room let in the sound of the restaurant crew preparing for the next morning's rations. Within a few hours, the smell of coffee drifted into the classroom. Dorothy's mind associated the aroma of a fresh brew with waking up, and she found it nearly impossible to sleep through the smell. She was tired and she was sick. Yet she was needed. Cobb had appointed herself director of the camp's nursing services. Dorothy was due every day at the infirmary. And, true to form, she went without complaint.

Within days of the nurses' arrival, devastating news crashed into the prison with one troubling announcement after the next. First the camp commander told the inmates the president of the Philippines was dead. Many of the inmates felt defeated—the country was without a leader. Others considered the source and distrusted the information. In truth, President Manuel Quezon was still alive, although he was afflicted with tuberculosis. Quezon evacuated to Australia and then on to the United States, where he continued his duties in exile.

A day after the fictitious Quezon announcement, the prison commander was pleased to report that General MacArthur had retreated to Australia in defeat. The inmates' reactions varied, and Americans expressed confidence in the Allied forces. MacArthur, they rationalized, had only left because he believed the United States was close to defeating Japan. But within a few weeks, the guards triumphantly circulated copies of the *Manila Tribune*, which showed a photograph of four army leaders negotiating the surrender of American and Filipino forces in Bataan.

In the photo, a colonel sat with his head in his hand. Next to him, General Edward P. King crossed his legs and leaned forward, looking anxious. The inmates scrutinized the photograph. Several prisoners were acquainted with General King, and the other inmates eagerly asked, do you think it's really him? The inmates who knew King admitted it appeared to be him in the photograph. But was he really surrendering? Or were they negotiating the terms of the Japanese surrender? Some argued that the latter seemed more likely.

The photograph was legitimate, as was the surrender in the Philippines. For months, the Japanese had strangled supply delivery, and American and Filipino forces were starved and weakened. General King trusted the surrender would save American lives. During the negotiations, King pressed for safe transport of military personnel to prisoner of war camps. He envisioned his tired men riding in buses or flat trucks. The Japanese did not honor the request. American and Filipino troops were forced to march more than sixty miles inland. The journey was later remembered as the Bataan Death March, in which one thousand American and nine thousand Filipino men died.

The fall of Bataan brought a new wave of inmates to Santo Tomas, most of them women and children who had been trapped in mountain towns or mining camps. They were starved, sick, and suffering from fresh emotional wounds. During their medical examinations, they confided in the nurses what they knew of the surrender. Dorothy listened with concern as they tearfully told of emaciated US forces, who lacked ammunition to fire at the enemy. Filipino civilians had eagerly shared supplies, but these provisions were soon depleted.

Dorothy ached for her fellow servicemen. She thought of the starving men in Bataan walking up to Japanese bayonets with their arms raised in surrender. And she shuddered over the mistreatment of her corpsmen, who she heard were now shut up in the prison in the former elementary school. But surely, she hoped, it would end soon. American forces were still hunkered down on the island of Corregidor.

For the next few weeks, the idea of a victory at Corregidor gave the prisoners hope and rumors gave them life. Someone had heard that the Japanese in Manila were boarding up their stores. They surmised the Japanese were leaving the city in preparation for an American invasion. Optimism swelled, leading some inmates to unrealistic conclusions. They decided the newspaper images of surrendering American forces were overblown. They believed it was probably true that *some* soldiers were captured but pointed out that the photographs showed only a couple dozen men with their arms raised. Cynical inmates listened to clandestine radios and discredited the optimists. They covertly tuned into broadcasts from San Francisco and heard the American announcers admit that US forces in Bataan had indeed surrendered.

Then, in early May, the guards proudly distributed copies of the *Manila Tribune* announcing the fall of Corregidor. The Allied forces were completely defeated in the Philippines. The members of the Japanese Imperial Army were now the ones surging with optimism. They believed they would conquer the mainland United States and dominate the world. A few inmates preserved hope and refused to believe the *Tribune* headline until one of the radio operators confirmed it was true. President Roosevelt had addressed the nation.

In front of the main building, Peg Nash found herself in the wrong place at the wrong time. In the two months the nurses had been in Santo Tomas, they had heard stories of the sentries' viciousness. In February, the guards claimed three inmates had escaped. The accusation was fairly sketchy, given that there was so much fluidity to the camp. Many inmates received day passes to leave the grounds for work or medical treatment. But the three men were apprehended outside the camp and dragged inside to the main building. For hours, the inmates heard the men scream in agony as they were beaten and tortured. Two days later, the men were brought to a grave site, shot, and buried in the shallow graves.

The torture and execution of the men was violence the inmates had only heard, but on other occasions they'd actually witnessed the same sort of unpredictable savagery. In January, the commander permitted a Filipino vendor to sell ice cream from a pushcart. For two days, he sold his products and then left quietly. On the third day, the guards waited until he sold his inventory, then repeatedly struck his face and stripped him of his earnings. Inmates holding ice cream stood paralyzed as the bloodied vendor stumbled from the camp. In the coming months, Japanese soldiers hauled Filipino citizens into the camp for beatings. Most of the victims were young men, who were strapped to trees and then brutally whipped in front of a crowd of stunned, wincing inmates.

Nurse Peg was near the main building when soldiers dragged in a young Filipino. They tied the panicked young man to a tree and began rounding up inmates to witness the assault. Peg was steered into the throng. Satisfied with the presence of the prisoners, the soldiers turned their attention to the victim. The inmates flinched and lowered their eyes as the soldiers pummeled the man. Many of the prisoners trembled and fought waves of nausea. The attack only seemed to intensify the longer it persisted. The soldiers raised their bayonets and directed the knifepoints at the victim's stomach. They took turns piercing the man's torso with the bayonets. Blood gushed from the wounds. The soldiers untied the nearly dead victim and dragged him from the camp. Once he was gone, the shaken witnesses were allowed to disperse.

Witnesses whispered accounts to confidants and described the anger they felt toward the soldiers. The killing gave them a new rage they'd never felt until they saw such atrocity. Peg, however, had seen savagery in her lifetime. In the wards at Cavite following the bombs, she'd felt the still artery of the little boy who died alone. In Santa Scholastica, she'd grimaced as sentries shadowboxed corpsmen and slapped physicians. And she knew she was once scheduled for execution after the patient escaped—Cobb had revealed the truth weeks later. The beating was one more terror Peg tried to bury deep, but she found it was easily disinterred. Asked years later about witnessing the beating, she simply said the guards did "terrible things in that camp."

———————

Lights-out was in effect. Dorothy lay in bed as Susie Pitcher wheezed in the cot next to her. Dorothy was accustomed to the noises in room 30A, and she was sleeping better. She was also learning to tolerate camp life—even the bathrooms, which were a source of shame that required months of adaptation. In the main building, women stood in lengthy lines to wash in the communal shower or relieve themselves in doorless stalls. Most followed the advice of a snappish sign that suggested, IF YOU WANT PRIVACY, CLOSE YOUR EYES. They also averted their eyes to avoid humiliating whoever found herself in a stall, faced with an audience. In the showers, however, it was impossible to grant one another privacy, as four or five women crowded naked under one showerhead to rinse off while others in line looked on.

The nurses had a few privileges that made camp life more livable. Because they worked four-hour shifts, they were not required to stand in the chow line, which typically took one hour of an inmate's time. The navy nurses were permitted to collect their rations directly from the kitchen and take their plates to a shanty Chief Nurse Cobb had secured. Inmates were required to eat outside, and the dining area was fly infested and repulsive. But those with a shanty had the privilege of taking their meals away from the clatter of the thousands of other inmates. To Dorothy, quietly eating in the shanty almost felt like a luxury.

Nurse Susie cared more for cigarettes than food. Her raspy breathing hinted at the extent of the damage to her lungs. She lay in bed, fighting to breathe. It took a moment for Dorothy to register a change in Susie's wheezing. The crackling breaths were suddenly labored, more desperate. Dorothy flipped over. Susie was sitting upright, clutching a pillow to her chest.

"This isn't emphysema," Susie gasped.

It was a heart attack. Dorothy summoned Cobb. The chief nurse pushed her way through the mosquito netting, calling for nurse Goldia O'Haver to assist her.

"Go back to bed," Cobb ordered Dorothy.

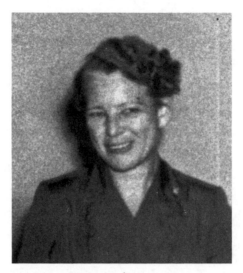

Navy nurse Susie Pitcher. *Courtesy of Bureau of Medicine and Surgery*

Cobb and Goldia helped Susie from her bed, navigating her down the narrow aisle and through the curtain blocking the doorway. Dorothy watched the women disappear behind the sheet and into the darkness. She sat on her bed and considered trying to sleep but felt too anxious. Being left behind made her feel both helpless and useless. Frustrated, she quietly crept from the room and into the dark stairwell. She lit a match, held it up to the cigarette pressed between her lips, and took a deep breath.

Being a prisoner of war meant never being alone but always being on your own. Dorothy and the other nurses were together constantly in the crowded camp, but they had to endure their own individual hardships. Susie recovered from her heart attack—and continued to smoke. Bertha Evans experienced abdominal pains and was sent to a Manila hospital for a hysterectomy. And Edwina Todd became increasingly weak. A camp physician informed Edwina that she should not expect to survive the war.

Edwina was surprised by the doctor's candor, especially since it was standard practice not to tell an ailing patient how long he or she might survive. Edwina questioned why the physician had told her. She was trapped in a prison camp—it wasn't as if she could seize the last few months of her life by visiting with friends or family.

Edwina suspected that part of her condition was related to malnutrition, and she might be able to heal herself if she could purchase supplemental food from the canteen. Each inmate received a small stipend, and Cobb was occasionally able to secure extra cash for her nurses. Neither was ever enough. However, the consumer economy that existed in Santo Tomas provided enterprising inmates with an income source. The hallways were jammed with vendors selling food and supplying services such as haircuts or clothes mending. Edwina noticed how no one had thought to lend or sell books.

Edwina saw opportunity in the inmates' daily boredom. She applied for a vendor's license and received the right to open the Anchor Library. The other nurses pooled together their books and solicited donations. In time, Edwina had more than two hundred books labeled with the signature blue anchor. Books were loaned out for five centavos per day, or twenty-five centavos per week. Edwina set up a table in one of the hallways. She mixed among the barbers, bakeshop goods, and candy makers. The other nurses took over the library during Edwina's frequent rest breaks. Receiving a cut of the income helped the women tolerate Edwina's bad moods.

Life fell into a rhythm of work, standing in line, retreating to the shanty, and feeling disappointed at mealtimes. For weeks, the nurses wondered about their army counterparts and whether they were surviving the war. They thought of Ann, who had left so eagerly for Bataan, and hoped she was alive.

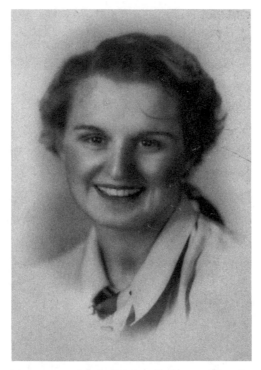

Navy nurse Carrie Edwina Todd. *Courtesy of Bureau of Medicine and Surgery*

In early July, an excited crowd brought Dorothy and a few other nurses to the front of the main building. A caravan had arrived carrying several dozen women. They were army nurses. The women appeared tired, dirty, and thin. They wearily faced the applauding crowd who welcomed them as heroes. Dorothy looked among the army nurses and registered a familiar face—Gwendolyn Henshaw from Los Angeles. The two women had attended nursing school together. Dorothy never knew Gwendolyn joined the army. She pushed through the crowd, eager to see a friend from home.

"Gwendolyn! Gwendolyn!" she called, waving her arm.

Gwendolyn started toward Dorothy. "Dottie?" she answered. "Dottie Still, is that really you?"

A guard stepped in front of the crowd and pushed everyone back. The army nurses were ordered into an old convent, segregated from the rest of the camp and forbidden to talk to anyone outside their group. The navy nurses assumed their army counterparts would be released after their belongings were thoroughly searched. But the women did not emerge from the brick building. The army women, the camp was informed, were in "quarantine." The inmates surmised it was because the army nurses could be plied for information.

By August, the army women were permitted to mix with the general camp population. At the hospital, army captain Maude Davison relieved Chief Nurse Cobb from her position as director of nursing services. Cobb acquiesced, rationalizing that the army's nursing corps was much larger. Cobb's civility, however, promptly dissolved when Davison posted a schedule and excluded all navy and civilian nurses from service. A terse conversation inspired Davison to rewrite a schedule that included both groups of military women.

Dorothy found the two military cultures distinct and well personified by their respective leaders. Davison was abrupt and loud. She pounded her fists on desks and physically demanded action. Cobb was quiet yet intimidating. As much as Dorothy hated to compliment her icy commander, she much preferred Cobb's style. She sensed the army nurses favored their own and considered Cobb a pushover.

Inmates also found the army nurses abrasive. One internee kept a secret diary, which included a chronology of events. He had recorded when the navy nurses arrived at the prison, describing them as "fine girls." When the army nurses arrived, he noted that only "some were nice."

Prisoner Margaret Sherk was also critical. Margaret and her young son David cycled from one illness to the next and depended on the nurses to keep them alive. She seemed to expect them to be like the sweet versions from home, who offered an extra pillow or scurried down the ward to bring a glass of water. The army nurses were war veterans, and they were painfully traumatized. Margaret and the other inmates had no sense of what the women had endured.

7

Where Were You
When We Needed Help?

DOROTHY RESTED UNDER a tree, absorbed in a book. In the nine months she'd been a prisoner of war, she found reading was the only way to truly escape. She didn't notice when army nurse Gwendolyn Henshaw sat down beside her. The two women greeted each other casually, as if they were back in Los Angeles and taking a break from the county hospital.

Until the day Gwendolyn arrived at the camp, the two hadn't seen each other since graduation, almost seven years earlier. Gwendolyn had been assigned to Sternberg Hospital and evacuated to Corregidor. Seeing each other again made them recall the younger versions of themselves. They spoke of life before the war and then carefully treaded into the topic of the December attacks. They found similarities in their nursing experiences after the bombing. The parallels ended as the army nurses evacuated to field hospitals and the navy nurses remained in Manila. It seemed to the army nurses as though the navy nurses intentionally sat out the battle.

"Where were you when we needed help?" Gwendolyn asked earnestly.

Dorothy assured Gwendolyn the navy nurses hadn't chosen to remain in Manila. Their orders to join the army nurses never came and they felt abandoned. But as Gwendolyn began describing the horrors of the past few months, Dorothy felt grateful the navy nurses hadn't experienced such trauma. At Corregidor, the US Army had maintained an elaborate labyrinth of tunnels under Malinta Hill. The bombproof tunnel spared the nurses the agony of a direct impact. Army nurses elsewhere, Gwendolyn revealed, were not as fortunate.

Nurses in Bataan had been separated to two field hospitals, and both were immediately overrun with casualties. There were more injured or ill men than beds. They also lacked mosquito nets, medical supplies, pharmaceuticals, and drinking water. As food stores dwindled, fearless nurses sampled boiled monkey and roasted rat. The wildlife learned to avoid the hungry humans and another food source was soon lost.

In early April, the Japanese bombers came for Hospital #1. Patients trapped in traction ropes shrieked and pleaded to be cut down. A priest prayed for the ward as patients rolled under their beds. One of the wards took a direct hit, and the force knocked the women to the ground. The nurses felt as though the pressure from the concussion were ripping their bodies apart. They staggered to their feet, struggling to breathe in a cloud of burning explosives. They instinctively inspected their own bodies for shrapnel wounds and contusions, and then set out to pull patients from the wreckage.

There were few survivors in that ward. The metal bed frames were twisted and speckled with flesh and blood. The tin roof was ripped from the building and the nurses saw that the bodies of decapitated men had been blasted into the jungle. They stared into the brush at the swinging limbs and unidentifiable torsos, looking for a hint of recognition. In the highest branches, they glimpsed tattered pajamas.

The nurses lived in the devastated field hospital for the next two days. They helped dig survivors out of the rubble. They paid their respects as bodies were buried in a mass grave. And they held the hands of dying men whose fearful eyes searched their faces for comfort.

Then, suddenly, evacuation orders came. The army nurses had thirty minutes to pack their belongings and board a bus for Corregidor. Bataan was falling, and the army was uncertain how the Japanese would treat female captives. The nurses protested against abandoning their patients and cried when they left their wounded. As the bus rumbled through the jungle, civilians banged on the windows and pleaded to come aboard. The nurses, already jarred by months of violence, were shaken by the fraught faces chasing the bus.

Within three weeks, the army nurses knew how the civilians had felt as the bus sped past and slipped from view. The Japanese had Corregidor surrounded. Twenty-two nurses were relieved of their assignments, and the women not chosen for evacuation would soon be prisoners of war. Envy and fear surged as the women destined for prison camps watched the evacuees pack small bags and head for an airfield. A few weeks later, another twelve nurses were selected for a submarine transport. Navy nurse Ann Bernatitus received evacuation orders. The short stick that sent Ann to Sternberg was the same one that brought her to the waterfront, where a submarine carried her to Australia.

Under the shade tree, Gwendolyn detailed these horrors for Dorothy, and she lost sight of her old friend as her memories became clear images in her mind. All the nurses experienced these types of flashbacks, which had the power to override what the eye saw and replace it with what the mind remembered. A nurse might be standing in the shower line or lying in bed when a memory rose up, bringing her back to a moment her mind refused to forget. A suffering patient. A limb dangling from a tree. Locking eyes with a frantic civilian chasing the bus. When a nurse's thoughts became ensnared with these mental pictures, she sometimes wondered whether they might point to a larger purpose behind all the horror. But the more a woman thought about such things, the more she realized there was no way to make sense of any of it.

As the year progressed, new arrivals learned that life at Santo Tomas was intentionally unstable and the Japanese Imperial Army rewrote rules on a whim. For example, the line for receiving packages from people on the outside was routinely shut down, and the guards threatened permanent closure. Inmates who depended on the packages fretted for their futures until the line suddenly reopened under new operating terms.

Camp leadership changed several times as well. The first commander had exhibited a viciousness more commonly seen in the prison camps reserved for soldiers. The camp's early arrivals were still shaken by the screams of the three escaped men who had been caught, ruthlessly beaten, and then executed. The second commander was a benign replacement. But the former diplomat was superseded in September by two English speakers, Aikida Kodaki and S. Kuroda. The inmates thought of Kodaki as belligerent. His counterpart, Kuroda, was seen as sympathetic but rash.

A clear double standard emerged. The camp rules were unpredictable, but the new commanders expected the executive committee to maintain strict order among the inmates. The commanders found fault in slight infractions. Every night, names of rule breakers were read over the loudspeaker along with their violations. Milder punishments ranged from a scolding to loss of privileges. The prison's jail was the worst punishment, and it resembled a monkey cage with a can for a toilet. Dorothy thought the idea of sending inmates to jail was ridiculous. They were *already* in prison.

The commanders mostly focused on inmates whose actions might cause visiting military or diplomatic officials to view the camp as poorly run. Inmates who were caught with alcohol or found to be intoxicated received jail sentences, whereas fighting among inmates was not a punishable offense. Such fights were typically resolved by room monitors or the executive committee. Stealing, refusal to work, and personal conflicts were also handled by the inmates' elected leaders.

Limiting male-female relations was among the commanders' top concerns. Men's and women's sleeping quarters were separate, even for married couples. But a few pregnancies revealed that couples had found private spaces to be together. After a few months, the guards realized the shanties were ideal places for amorous inmates to connect. The commander ordered immediate removal of the front and the back doors, which allowed any passersby to look inside the little huts. Truly motivated couples simply took their rendezvous into the shadows of

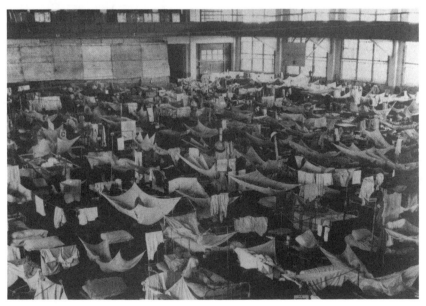

Sleeping quarters for men in a gymnasium at Santo Tomas. *Courtesy of US Army*

the camp. But most inmates actually lost their drive for sex. Men whispered their concerns to the camp doctors and received assurances that it was normal under such conditions to temporarily lose sexual function.

By late October, inmates craved a diversion. Although Christmas was months away, it held the promise of distraction. Christmas preparation groups formed, and the inmates strategized to ensure every child received a toy on Christmas morning. Inmates with carpentry abilities turned scrap wood into doll beds or toy trains. Those with sewing skills stitched rag dolls with matching outfits. Others turned their attention to holiday festivities. A children's choir practiced songs for a brief holiday program, and an adult group planned a full choral performance. The camp's theater society decided to mount a performance of *A Christmas Carol*.

The two commanders tolerated the Christmas preparations, as it served their purpose. Several Red Cross agencies were sniffing around the prison, eager to distribute relief kits. Allowing the inmates to celebrate their holiday season gave the appearance the prisoners were in good health and well cared for. By early December, the commanders also felt obligated to accept a donation from the South African Red Cross. Dorothy gathered with the crowd to watch the supplies being delivered. The inmates stared eagerly as three thousand pounds of sugar were unloaded from the truck. Dorothy looked at the sugar bags with apprehension. The amount was indeed tremendous, but Dorothy considered the larger context. There were three thousand inmates at the camp, and she had to quietly admit the possibility they might be imprisoned indefinitely. How long would this truly last them?

Dorothy had more enthusiasm when the Red Cross delivered individual "comfort kits." Every inmate received four eight-ounce cans of corned beef. There were also small tins containing bacon, chocolate cake, cheese, condensed milk, crackers, crushed tomatoes, margarine, marmalade, meat spread, pudding, sugar, and tea. Dorothy felt the comfort kits delivered a reminder that the inmates were remembered by the outside world. But others felt sickened, as if the kits were taunting them with a taste of all they were missing.

To inmate Abraham Hartendorp, a Colorado magazine publisher who was nearing his fiftieth birthday, the kits were demoralizing. Getting excited about a tin of pudding or meat spread felt humiliating to a man of his distinction. He wrote in his secret diary that he pitied inmates who lost self-control and ate most of their kits' contents in one sitting. And he felt a quiet irritation as engineers, bankers, corporate executives—people who'd once had pride—debated whether to open a margarine packet or save it for later. It all seemed so *pathetic*, he thought.

Christmas in the camp began on December 22 as the adult choir performed its holiday concert with a program of Christmas carols. Dorothy sat in the crowd, thinking of how the holiday had new meaning for her. Dorothy had converted to Catholicism on Easter Sunday, with nurse Peg Nash as her godmother. Her new faith, Dorothy felt, gave her a sense of belonging. She was also more emotionally prepared to face the possibility that she might die young. It was a morbid thought, and Dorothy feigned sanguinity among other inmates. She readily agreed when other inmates claimed, "Forty-three and we'll be free!" But in her quiet moments, she stopped looking forward. The future was too volatile and all her previous attempts to predict their liberation had ended in disappointment. Each shattered timeline cracked her resolve, leaving her with a sense of hopelessness.

Dorothy did not want to risk being broken. As a nurse, she was needed by thousands of inmates who saw her uniform and felt deep reassurance. Anyone who was sick and admitted into the makeshift hospital found they were not alone. They had the nurses, who were the anchors of the camp. These anchors kept morale from drifting, which was not easy in a place where desperate adults squeezed margarine packets into their mouths to give a quick boost to their fat-deprived bodies. But at times anchors need to be lifted up, and Dorothy found pleasure in the Christmas carol performance. She listened placidly as the choir sang familiar songs that reminded her of past Christmases and her life before the war. The last song of the evening, "Silent Night," brought the audience a momentary sense of calm.

The next day brought a moment of humor. The camp commanders allowed the inmates to view a Hollywood film. But first they played a propaganda film that showed Japanese children engaged in various sports. The guards were proud of the film and without irony urged the inmates not to interrupt with applause. The inmates were not impressed with the "sport show." They gave each other cautious, sideways glances as they watched the children on-screen perform calisthenics and kick rolling balls. A narrator with a childish voice described the country's supposed dominance, which caused inmates to roll their eyes. At the end of the film, the children paraded with torches while the phrase "Toward a Free Asia" flashed on the screen. The movie dramatically concluded with a close-up of a burning torch. The inmates choked back laughter. The filmmaker had attempted to create a symbolic conclusion, but instead gave the image of Japan on fire. Inmates later agreed they very much liked that thought.

The 1941 film *The Feminine Touch* followed. It told the story of an American college professor who writes a book about marital jealousy, despite having no idea whenever another man notices his wife. Early in the film, the professor and his wife travel to New York City to meet his publisher. The publisher falls for the professor's wife, while his comely assistant takes an interest in the professor. In the antics that follow, the professor finally burns with jealousy. Inmate Abraham Hartendorp disliked the film and made careful note in his diary that the movie was second rate. The characters' problems were self-imposed and trivial to prisoners of war. But Abraham, like so many other inmates, was riveted by the images of the outside world. He was particularly interested in seeing the scenes in which the actors dined at clean tables and slept in rooms not crammed with hundreds of cots.

The guards allowed more programming on Christmas Eve as both the children's choir and the theater society performed. On Christmas Day, a priest performed an open-air mass, and the homemade gifts were distributed to the children of the camp. The big boon, however, was the announcement that comfort kits had arrived from the Canadian Red Cross. Anticipation spread as the inmates imagined lathering themselves with soap or shaving cream. People thought of the luxury that would come with the "toilet kit," which for a short time would enhance the scant five-square ration of toilet tissue they received each day.

The commanders proved to be in no hurry to distribute the goods, and the packages languished for weeks in the gymnasium. It was almost as if the men in charge gauged the camp morale to be too high after the Christmas holiday. But there was another reason for the delay. The executive committee realized the camp had a dwindling supply of condensed milk to distribute to the children. They estimated the supply would deplete within five months, and they considered opening the comfort kits and confiscating the condensed milk they contained.

The other inmates, particularly the Americans, seethed. The executive committee had no right to "loot" the parcels the Canadian Red Cross had intended for each inmate to receive. Furthermore, what was the executive committee implying when they said the milk supply would deplete in five months? That they would still be prisoners in five months' time? American inmates scoffed at the unpatriotic implication. They felt it was disloyal to suggest that the US and Filipino forces needed more than a few months to retake the islands. These inmates were angry that the executive committee did not share their optimism and wondered what had happened to "Forty-three and we'll be free."

Part III

1943

8

Fed Up with the Way Things Have Been Going

DOROTHY STOOD IN the lobby of the main building, near the command-ers' office. A worried crowd was forming outside the closed door, wondering if the rumors were true. The nurse searched the anxious swarm trying to find a former patient she remembered from her San Diego days. The man was a marine who did not evacuate Manila and was taken prisoner along with the civilians. The Japanese had forgot-ten about him and some thirty other members of the armed services. Many of the men had wives and children in the camp, and none were eager to correct the oversight.

After a year of internment, one angry soldier had betrayed the entire group. R. J. Owens was not getting along with his room monitor, nor the other men in his dormitory. He began using an empty stairwell landing as his personal space. Bunking on the land-ing was forbidden, and the executive committee ordered him to move. R.J. threatened to complain to the camp commanders, and the executive committee fired back with the same warning. They did not anticipate that he would expose himself and the other enlisted men.

The next day, the commander ordered all active members of the Allied armed forces to report to his office. The entire camp was stunned by the betrayal, and R.J. was confronted by inmates who demanded to know why he had turned on his fellow prisoners, especially since there was no reward for snitching—R.J. wouldn't be compensated with extra rations or a better sleeping arrangement. Instead, he and the other enlisted men were at risk for severe punishment.

R.J. remained unapologetic when confronted. "I'm fed up with the way things have been going," he barked back.

The enlisted men and their loved ones spent a miserable night, wondering if the next day meant separation or even execution. The Japanese army held a clear and cold distinction between civilian and military prisoners. Anyone taken captive "while still able to resist" was considered a criminal whose offenses were punishable by death. Inmates feared the enlisted men would be executed for concealing their military affiliation. Others thought the men would be sent to a military prison camp, where the dire conditions meant a low chance of survival.

Dorothy watched the enlisted men glumly enter the commanders' office to identify themselves. The men were well liked among the inmates. One was an amiable room monitor. A few played in the prison's baseball league. Several were part of the evening broadcasts the commanders permitted over the loudspeaker.

Dorothy spotted the marine she had known in San Diego. "I can't begin to tell you how sorry I am," she consoled.

"I'm sorry too, ma'am," he answered.

The marine and the other men were ordered to the front of the building. Dorothy tensed as the front gates opened to accept a large flatbed truck. Hundreds of people watched apprehensively as the thirty enlisted men stepped forward. The sentry assigned to the transport directed them to leave behind their bedrolls and bags. Money was forbidden, so the men faced friends in the crowd and flung their coins. Their nervous eyes lingered on the familiar faces.

As the engine started, a Japanese civilian emerged from the commanders' office and climbed into the passenger seat. "Don't worry," the civilian shouted toward the crowd. "They will come back. You will have to trust us."

The truck rumbled away. The stunned crowd was still. The unnerving sound of a sobbing woman broke the quiet. The woman was married to one of the enlisted men and they had a three-month-old baby. She had arrived too late to say good-bye and she wept in utter distress. The anguish unfolded through the crowd. Children whimpered. Adults sickened by the agony wiped away tears.

It felt like a death, the type that came from an unforeseen accident in which all was well in one moment and then shattered in the next. A former member of the executive committee was compelled to plead for leniency. He explained to Commander Kuroda how the thirty men had never concealed their military status. Almost all entered the camp wearing their military uniforms, and the previous commanders were well aware of their presence. Kuroda claimed he was convinced by the appeal and would try to prevent any unjust punishment. The next day, Kuroda demanded that all civilian men employed by the military as noncombatants register at his office. About 250 men complied. But the men were never questioned further, nor transferred from the camp. The inmates wondered, *What did that mean?*

The inmates did not know what would happen to the enlisted men either. The Japanese civilian had assured the crowd the men were safe, and Kuroda had promised to intercede against harsh punishment. But the inmates knew better than to trust their captors. And because another inmate had snitched to the commander, the prisoners now knew they could not trust each other.

———————

Trust was a question even among the nurses. The navy nurses had faith in one another, and the army nurses were confident in their own. But could the two groups trust each other? Dorothy had noticed from the outset how the nursing corps' cultures were distinct, yet they worked alongside each other in the makeshift hospital, tending to about one hundred patients. Some of the patients were recovering from cardiac events that were no doubt induced by the stress of their captivity. Others had infectious diseases such as the flu, bacillary and amoebic dysentery, and dengue fever. In the tuberculosis ward, the nurses cared for inmates who had received chest X-rays at a local hospital, as well as a recommendation to remain in bed for up to a year. The nurses also managed outpatient cases, mostly people suffering from vitamin deficiencies. They drained boils, cleaned open wounds, and looked at swollen, red gums. They advised women whose menstrual cycles became heavy and constant, and those who had stopped menstruating completely.

Not all the ailments were physical. There were inmates who alternated between a depressive comatose state and hysterical weeping. The physicians dosed extreme cases with sedatives, and the subdued patients stared blankly at the ceiling, failing to notice when a nurse brought a glass of water or ran a wet sponge down their arm. The most mentally debilitated patients were deemed "psychopaths" and transferred to outside institutions; their subsequent fates were unknown.

Tensions increased as the camp grew ever more overcrowded. As the Japanese military imprisoned more mothers with children, the area set aside for them started to seem inadequate. The executive committee sought out a larger space and ultimately proposed designating "the big house"—the old convent where the army nurses lived—for this purpose. The army nurses refused. They had no interest in relinquishing the privacy of the convent and moving into the lice-infested main building. An uncomfortable negotiation began, and the executive committee threatened to move the women's belongings. The army nurses plotted a response.

A strike had potential. If the army nurses didn't show up for their shifts, the hospital would have to scramble to fill the void with civilian and navy nurses. Coverage was possible in the short term, but the patient population would soon overwhelm the temporary staff, and the executive committee would have to reconsider. The idea, however, posed substantial risks. The nurses might lose the standoff and find themselves in a worse position, for both their living quarters and their work detail. All inmates were required to work, and the laid-off civilian nurses were relegated to kitchen chores.

The *threat* of a strike seemed more promising. The women considered how best to relay the information and decided it should be passed from one nurse to the next—army nurse to navy nurse, friend to friend. The strike planners targeted Dorothy, urging her friend Gwendolyn to quietly share the women's interest in striking. Gwendolyn approached Dorothy the day after the enlisted men were forced onto the flatbed truck. Distrust blanketed the camp, and people were uneasy. When Gwendolyn whispered to her friend that the army nurses intended to strike, Dorothy was stunned. She'd never heard of nurses going on strike and leaving their patients.

"You can't do that," Dorothy protested.

Gwendolyn claimed the plan was in place. Starting the next morning, the army nurses would not show up for work. Dorothy was haunted by the revelation. She wanted to tell Chief Nurse Cobb but hesitated to betray her friend's confidence. She approached Cobb in the navy nurses' shanty and in a roundabout way asked her superior to schedule her for the next day. Cobb was suspicious, especially because Dorothy knew she had no say in the schedule. With a bit of prodding, Dorothy disclosed the details of the strike.

The next morning, Dorothy was at the hospital, ready to assume a shift. She was surprised to see Gwendolyn dressed and ready to work. Gwendolyn revealed that Cobb had reported the strike, which prompted the executive committee to seek a compromise with the army nurses. The women would indeed move to the main building, but they would have their own quarters, including a room they could use as a dining room. Although they would have to share the bathroom facilities with the other women in the building, the army nurses considered the new facilities an upgrade from their space in the convent and agreed to the move.

Gwendolyn was pleased with the outcome. She was friendly when Dorothy approached her with an apology.

"That's OK," Gwendolyn said brightly. She admitted she'd used her friend to advance their interests. "We were counting on you to talk."

Betrayal, vermin, and disease crawled through the camp, as did depression. The inmates painfully missed their former lives. Young people felt that the trajectory of their lives had been unfairly derailed. Nurses Peg Nash and Mary Chapman were supposed to be newlyweds celebrating their first wedding anniversaries with the men they loved. Instead of pulling their cake tops out of the freezer, they were unmarried and living in a bedbug-infested dormitory. Dorothy noticed times when Peg needed space to grieve. Peg's bed was at the end of the room, and her only privacy was to lie on her side and face the wall. Dorothy and the other nurses knew not to bother Peg when they found her this way.

Mary's thoughts dwelled on her own love story, which had a biting twist that she confronted in her quiet moments. She would clutch two knitting needles and mechanically loop and pull string. Her vacant expression indicated she had gone into a trance no one dared to disrupt. Before her engagement, Mary had extended her tour in the Philippines so she could stay close to her fiancé. But he was injured in the attack on Cavite and evacuated before the Japanese entered Manila. He was safely back in the United States, and Mary was trapped in a prison camp.

They all had coping mechanisms. Nurse Eldene Paige propped herself on her bed and wrote poetry in a notebook. Dietitian Bertha Evans muffled her anxieties during the day, and then lay awake at night, wondering when she might see liberation. She thought back to the boat ride to Hawaii when an officer had warned her she would be eating fish heads and rice before the war was over. Fish heads no longer sounded like a threat but seemed like an excellent source of vitamins and fatty acids. It was hard to think about how much they'd lost and how profoundly they'd changed.

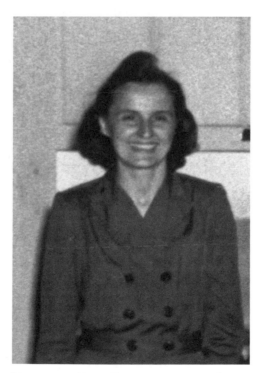

Navy nurse Mary Chapman. *Courtesy of Bureau of Medicine and Surgery*

Other inmates endured recurring bouts of insomnia, particularly when the cruelty of the camp picked at their minds and kept them up at night. Toward the end of January, the commander ordered all pregnant women to identify themselves. Because sex was forbidden, the women and their male partners were subject to punishment. The women avoided naming their partners, but four men were identified and sentenced to jail terms. All the expectant mothers were ordered into confinement at a local hospital, and buses promptly rolled into the camp to service the transfer. Inmates were traumatized as they watched sobbing children pried from their mothers' arms.

At the end of the month, a former agony revisited the inmates. Four of the enlisted men who had been taken away were returned to the camp after proving they'd been discharged prior to the war. After being gone just a few weeks, the men were gaunt and pale, but they were alive. They came back with limited information: The Japanese army had not executed the enlisted men. Instead, they accepted the situation as a misunderstanding and sent the men to POW camps reserved for military. This news was highly distressing. The Santo Tomas inmates knew that prisoners in the military camps faced disease, advanced starvation, and daily violence. Family members pumped the four returning men for information, but they waved off questions. The commanders had warned them not to talk about their experiences, and the men did not want to risk disobeying their orders. Others in the camp had proved they could not be trusted.

9

They Will Suffocate!

BY MAY, INMATES began to worry about the upcoming typhoon season. Life in the camp was already uncertain, and people dreaded the unpredictable summer storms. Inmates who had built shanties traded ideas on how to protect against fierce winds or flooding. Although May was typically a quiet month for typhoons, the inmates instinctively sensed that an intense force was about to slam into the camp.

A disturbance was indeed brewing. In the first week of May, the inmates learned that Japanese premier Hideki Tōjō was visiting Manila. They were confused as to why the humorless leader was in the country, although a few events supplied a vague idea. The Japanese declared May 6 "Thanksgiving Day" and expected the Filipino people to give thanks to Japan. At a Manila parade ground, soldiers drafted Filipinos into a celebration in which they were required to bow deeply in the direction of Japan and observe a moment of silence for the Japanese war dead. The next day, the Japanese proclaimed May 7 a national holiday to celebrate the one-year anniversary of the fall of Corregidor.

The inmates speculated that Tōjō—who served as both the premier and minister of war—was in the country to pressure the Filipino leadership to declare themselves an enemy of the United States. Among the Americans, the patriotic hopeful argued Tōjō realized his country would soon lose the war and was looking for damage control by enlisting the support of the Filipino people.

The camp commanders were also uncertain about Tōjō's visit, and they wore their formal uniforms in case he stopped by without forewarning. Tōjō did not bother with Santo Tomas, nor did he pay much attention to the prisoners of war and the atrocities they suffered. While in Manila, he consulted the chief of staff for the Japanese army and received assurances that the rumors regarding the Bataan Death March had been overblown. Tōjō did not ask further questions, and left prisoner treatment to his subordinates.

His presence, however, had an impact on Santo Tomas. For months, the Japanese army had discussed shifting the entire camp into the countryside. The premier's visit prompted the commanders to expedite the move. They were not happy that the camp was on display to the Filipino people or that the locals had proved to be such a disruption, sharing food and medicine with the inmates and ferrying in secret notes that made intercamp communication possible.

Three days after "Thanksgiving Day," the public address system crackled to life and one of the commanders ordered the inmates to listen. In English, he announced that he had important news and planned to repeat his message twice. The internees stopped what they were doing. Women standing by the washtubs in the courtyard stood with suds in their hair. The nurses in the hospital paused quietly alongside patient beds. And people in the dormitories hushed each other and looked up toward the speakers. The commander explained that he had chosen a new location for a second camp: the University of the Philippines College of Agriculture, located about forty miles to the south in Los Baños. The campus was near Laguna de Bay, the largest freshwater lake in the islands. The commander called it an "ideal health resort" that would appeal greatly to the inmates.

Inmates exchanged glances. *Ideal health resort?* They were doubtful. The commander promised fresh air and vegetable gardens, which the inmates would be allowed to cultivate themselves. But the campus was not ready to receive the entire inmate population. The commander asked for eight hundred able-bodied men to volunteer to construct barracks and install a sanitation system. The commander was clear—if he did not promptly have the names of eight hundred volunteers, then he expected the executive committee to make selections.

Many inmates thought the commander's "health resort" claims were ridiculous. Some suspected that he was simply trying to trick the prisoners into entering a mass grave. Others worried about isolation from loved ones or the package line. In the next few hours, instead of volunteering, inmates sought out members of the executive committee and aggressively petitioned to remain in Santo Tomas. Men who were well-known bachelors claimed to have families in Manila whom they'd never mentioned before. Some showed medical statements diagnosing them as unfit for labor. One young man reported to the hospital with vomiting and debilitating stomach cramps. A medical inquiry revealed that he had conspired with his girlfriend to drink soapy water in order to elicit a coveted doctor's note.

Only two hundred men volunteered by the end of the evening, and the executive committee members were not keen to force another six hundred to transfer. In an attempt to convince the executive committee to assign the transfers, the commanders ordered three members to tour the new camp. The men made the trip within a day and reported back that the water supply at Los Baños was alarmingly inadequate. During the rainy season, the camp reservoir held fifty thousand gallons. If the camp reached its capacity of seven thousand people—as the Japanese army intended—then they would need three hundred thousand gallons daily to supply the camp's needs.

Concerned inmates waited in the lobby as the committee members shut the door to the commanders' office and tried to persuade their captors to cancel the transfer. From the lobby, prisoners heard the commanders' angry response. The defeated executive committee members retreated from the office to draw up a list of six hundred able-bodied men.

Dorothy looked up as the auburn-haired nurse sped in her direction. Mary Rose Harrington was on a mission to assemble the navy nurses. "Cobb wants us in the shanty right away," Mary Rose said urgently.

The meeting had to happen immediately. The list of inmates who would be transferred to Los Baños was forming, and civilian physician Dr. Charles N. Leach had asked Cobb if the navy nurses were willing to join him. It was not an easy assignment to accept. The twelve nurses would be the only women in a camp of 788 men. They would be responsible for providing medical care to the entire prison population under conditions Cobb could not predict. Los Baños was a gamble. There might be fresh air and the opportunity to grow vegetables. Or there might be starvation and a perilously low water supply. The building conditions were unknown, as was the temperament of the guards. At Santo Tomas, the guards typically minded the perimeter and ignored the inmates within. The nurses were not eager to relive their experiences at Santa Scholastica, where the sentries had been allowed to torment the women and slap the men.

The nurses were desperately needed. If the navy women were unwilling to go, then Leach would have to engage inexperienced volunteers. Captain Davison had made it clear that the army nurses were going to remain as one unit at Santo Tomas. Most of the civilian nurses did not want to go, as many had significant others in Santo Tomas or in nearby Bilibid Prison. Although Cobb felt she could not answer on behalf of her nurses, she wanted the transfer. Conditions at Santo Tomas were deteriorating. Food rations were down to two meals a day, and the breakfast cereal was typically infested with worms. Hygiene was difficult to maintain, and bedbugs and lice were so widespread that inmates no longer noticed as their fingers traveled across their skin in a constant itch.

With the women gathered in the shanty, Cobb made her case. "How do you feel about this?" she asked.

Dorothy hesitated. Santo Tomas was not ideal, but it was familiar. She had a routine. Every morning the guards played music over the loudspeakers to wake the camp. She waited in the toilet line, and then collected her meager breakfast from the kitchen. She worked a four-hour shift or busied herself with survival chores. The nurses knitted, sewed, and tried to extend the lifespan of fading clothing. They traded reading material, sometimes finding a magazine that was so old it felt fresh. Dorothy hated to forfeit the familiar. Yet she could not deny that she was needed elsewhere.

Refusal was an option. Dorothy was under no obligation to remain under Cobb's authority. The men in the prisoner of war camps were not maintaining rank, and the nurses were not responsible for continuing their duties in the medical corps. But their services would be far more valuable at Los Baños than they were at Santo Tomas, where the most serious cases were farmed out to local hospitals. In Los Baños, they would not have external hospitals to provide surgeries and support. The twelve nurses and two doctors would be responsible for all medical care, including surgery.

Cobb went around the shanty asking each nurse whether she would volunteer to go. Bertha Evans was a yes. Nurse anesthetist Susie Pitcher agreed. Surgical nurse Goldia O'Haver gave her consent. Peg Nash was willing. Mary Chapman wanted to go. Basilia Steward Torres, Mary Rose Harrington, Eldene Paige, Helen Gorzelanski, Edwina Todd—all said they were in.

Cobb looked at Dorothy.

"Yes," Dorothy agreed.

It was unanimous.

———————————

Dorothy woke suddenly. It was only 5:00 AM—an hour before inmates were usually expected to rise. The loudspeakers blared music, a clear indication the guards wanted the camp up early. It was a dreadful day for many women in the camp. They awoke with the knowledge that their husbands or boyfriends were being sent forty miles away into the unknown. They did not know when they would see each other next, or if they would ever meet again.

Margaret Sherk was one of the miserable women. She had been separated from her husband in the army. Now she would be losing her boyfriend, Chicagoan Gerald Sams, who had worked as a radio operator at Cavite.

In captivity at Santo Tomas, Gerald had proven himself profoundly resourceful with his repair skills and nesting instincts. He and Margaret started out as friends, and Gerald helped to make internment more bearable for Margaret and her young son. Margaret had been shaken when Gerald was drafted to Los Baños, and she felt as though her lifeline was severed. But the separation would prove to be advantageous. After his departure, Margaret realized she was pregnant with Gerald's child. Since reproduction was forbidden, his absence spared him from a thirty-day sentence in the prison's jail.

The women left behind at Santo Tomas were not the only ones feeling anxious. The transferring prisoners felt apprehensive about surrendering their baggage. Dorothy had turned over her belongings to the guards the previous day and then worried she'd unwittingly forfeited her property for good. Her possessions had dwindled down to a few precious items, barely more than an empty tin can and a bar of soap she'd saved from a comfort kit. But these items were not easy to replace, and Dorothy thought there was a strong possibility she might never see them again.

Dorothy tried to look forward. She collected her small handbag, which she was told she'd be allowed to carry aboard the train to Los Baños. She ducked under the mosquito net, walked down the narrow aisle, and passed through the curtain hanging in the doorway, leaving room 30A for the last time. With the other navy nurses, she joined the throng of inmates gathered in front of the main building. The atmosphere was tense with emotion. Apprehensive men were encouraged by friends who came to shake their hands and wish them well. Couples facing separation exchanged farewells and tried to comfort each other.

Distressed inmates cried as the trucks entered the front gate and sputtered down the long drive. The men went first, and the crowd thinned as hundreds of prisoners were hustled onto the open-air trucks. Women waved at their departing spouses until they were driven from view. Several of the wives approached the navy nurses and asked them to take care of their husbands until they were reunited. The army nurses also came to say good-bye and let their navy counterparts know they had been appreciated at Santo Tomas. Dorothy saw Gwendolyn among the army women and the two approached each other. Dorothy had long forgiven Gwendolyn for setting her up during the strike threat, and the two friends gave each other a tight hug.

"If the war ends before we get to Los Baños, I'll see you in the States," Gwendolyn assured Dorothy.

As the navy nurses waited to board their transport, Dorothy looked over at her chief nurse. Cobb was wearing a large army nurse uniform. The nurses' records were tucked around her waist, and she had again donned a lei to disguise the bulge. Dorothy followed Cobb into the back of their truck. Looking out, she saw a mass of people clapping their hands and cheering them on. The navy nurses looked at each other, some a bit surprised by the expression of appreciation. Were the inmates really cheering for them? And then they heard it, coming through the loudspeakers—a recording of their march song.

"*Stand Navy down the field, sails set to the sky . . .*"

The sound of horns and boisterous singing mixed in with the applauding crowd.

"*. . . Roll up the score, Navy, Anchors Aweigh.*"

Several of the nurses began to cry. They had indeed been anchors, but their commitment to nursing was something they'd felt compelled to do. They didn't realize anyone else had noticed.

———————

Dorothy climbed from the truck, holding her handbag as well as her food ration for the day—a boiled duck egg, a slice of bread, and a small bottle of water. As she approached the tracks, she was stunned to see a line of steel boxcars connected to a steaming locomotive. She looked down the track to see if there was another locomotive with passenger cars attached, but this was the only train on the tracks. It seemed implausible to Dorothy. Even *cattle* traveled in ventilated box-cars. These were shipping containers not meant for living creatures.

Nurse Peg Nash had the same reaction. *Surely*, Peg thought, *they are not going to put us in a boxcar.*

In a sealed boxcar, the prisoners would breathe in oxygen and release carbon dioxide, which would rapidly poison them all. And it would be a miserable death in which they all hyperventilated until they submitted to either unconsciousness or a choking sensation. Were the guards trying to kill them? Or did they not realize the potential for suffocation?

The nurses watched with growing concern as sentries divided the men and ordered them to load themselves into the cars. As the car filled, the men were pushed back to make room for more bodies.

The nurses saw that the inmates inside were standing shoulder to shoulder. The prisoners looked helplessly back at the nurses as the guards slammed the doors shut.

"They will suffocate!" Chief Nurse Cobb called out in a panic.

Cobb shoved her way to the two physicians who were waiting with the nurses. Dorothy watched as the two medical men approached the lieutenant in charge and explained how the sealed container meant certain death. The lieutenant relented, but only slightly. The side doors could be opened a crack to allow for fresh air once the train got moving. But the doors had to remain shut and locked until they left city limits.

The guards broke the nurses into pairs and ordered the women to walk to the front of the line. Starting with the first car, they directed two women to climb aboard each car. The women sensed they were being separated with a clear purpose—if anyone on their car escaped, then the two nurses would be executed as punishment. Dorothy and Helen Gorzelanski were each lifted into the same boxcar.

Dorothy turned and looked through the car. The men in the back appeared in shadows and silhouettes. They were packed so tightly that it was difficult to see where one body ended and the next began. Dorothy peered at the guards below as they heaved the door shut. She heard the clanking of an iron padlock secured in place. The train whistle blew several times and then the car lurched forward and jolted until it gained momentum and rolled from the train station. The train was not as they expected, and Dorothy had to wonder whether the "health resort" was in actuality a death camp.

———————————

The doors remained locked as the train wound its way out of the city limits. The day's outdoor temperature was in the nineties, and the heat in the boxcar soared past one hundred degrees. The hot air was suffocating, and the prisoners began to sweat profusely. They stood in the dark, feeling the movements of the train and wondering if the air supply would last to the city limits. The train eventually slowed and jerked to a halt. The padlock shackle clanged as it was pulled from the iron hasp, and bright sunlight suddenly hit the front of the car. Dorothy and Helen stood near the door, uncertain what to do.

"You girls sit here," one of the inmates suggested.

The door was open just wide enough for the women to sit with their legs hanging over the side of the car. It was a generous offer—they would be the only people on the car able to sit and feel the wind when the train picked up speed. Dorothy and Helen sat in the door frame, their legs pressed against each other as they squeezed into the space. The boxcar heaved forward, and Dorothy expected the train to increase in speed, but it chugged along slowly. Then the train unexpectedly stopped, waited, and allowed another train to speed past. The prisoners realized that what should have been a two-hour trip was going to take the better part of the day. The men in the back of the cars burned with heat, and their small water bottles were soon empty.

In another boxcar, Chief Nurse Cobb and Mary Rose pressed together. The inmates had debated how to equitably share the fresh air. Mary Rose offered her hat to be used as a type of wind scoop. It was the style of hat typically worn by Filipina women as sun protection, resembling a large, flat disk with a small indent for the head. The inmates took turns standing by the door and using the hat to fan the air. In Dorothy's car, the prisoners decided to rotate every twenty minutes so that each man had a chance to stand near the open door. At the suggestion, Dorothy and Helen rose to rotate to the back of the car, but the other inmates insisted the women remain seated at the door.

Dorothy returned to her seat on the ledge and watched the landscape slowly roll past. The train made her think about where she had been. She thought of her parents in Long Beach and worried her capture would cause them great stress. Her mind went back to her leave during Christmas 1939. She had her orders for the Philippines and her mother sensed the danger on the horizon. Throughout the visit, Arissa pleaded with Dorothy, saying, "Don't go." Defying orders was not an option, and Dorothy tried to assuage her mother's worries with assurances that she would return within two years. Now, she was seventeen months past the date of her promised return. And the transfer to Los Baños indicated she was sinking deeper into captivity. Liberation, Dorothy realized, was not coming anytime soon.

10

Take Them Outside

THE TRAIN SHRIEKED to a halt, and the guards ordered their human cargo to unload. Dorothy pushed herself from the side of the boxcar and merged with the streams of prisoners fleeing the intense heat. The mass of inmates trudged down the platform as the guards roared at the men to begin marching. Anyone who strayed from the pack in search of a water spigot was met with a bayonet point.

The nurses were separated from the men and loaded into the back of a coal-fueled truck. The soldier assigned to the truck sneered as the women placed their handbags on the cargo bed and hoisted themselves up. Mary Rose thought back to all the belligerent soldiers she had seen in the past two years and felt that the scowling man was the angriest she had ever seen. The soldier was enraged by what he perceived was the low-level assignment of guarding mere women. Sensing the conflict, about half a dozen male inmates climbed into the truck. The soldier's disposition improved immediately. If the women weren't so dehydrated, they might have cried from the degradation.

The truck's engine roared like a small plane and coughed black smoke into the air. As it sputtered from the station, Dorothy watched the procession of tired men fade from view. The truck picked up speed, whipping an appreciated breeze. Dorothy braced herself against the side as they descended into a green valley. A view of fruit trees and lush vegetation was quickly replaced with the familiar sight of imprisonment. The garrison assigned to Los Baños had already rimmed the campus with barbed wire and built an imposing guard tower near the back gate.

The truck creaked over a wooden bridge, and Dorothy looked down at the rippling stream that flowed beneath. In comparison to Santo Tomas, the new camp struck Dorothy as beautiful. Leafy trees surrounded part of the campus, and monkeys playfully swung from the branches. As the truck drove deeper into the compound, Dorothy saw a baseball diamond, soccer field, and bandstand. There was also a large gymnasium surrounded by a soft green lawn. Construction materials lined the perimeter, and she sensed the wide-open spaces would soon be filled with hastily made barracks and shanties.

The marching men had a three-mile distance to cover, and the women were directed to wait for the other inmates to arrive. Excitement briefly swelled when a guard passed each woman a drinking cup. The women hoped for water but received sake instead. Rather than feeling defeated, one of the nurses raised her cup in a toast. The other women clinked their cups together and smiled miserably.

A flashbulb burst. The women turned to see a guard holding a camera. Peg Nash knew what he was doing—snapping a photograph to wrongly claim the prisoners were treated fairly. Back at Santo Tomas, another guard had hunted her for days. He would follow her around the prison until she slipped into the safety of a crowded room. Peg feared he intended to rape her. Then one day in the ward, as she held a washbasin in her hands and listened sympathetically to a British patient, the stalking guard suddenly produced a camera and captured the image. Years later, Peg learned the photograph was used by the Japanese Imperial Army to assert that the prisoners were well

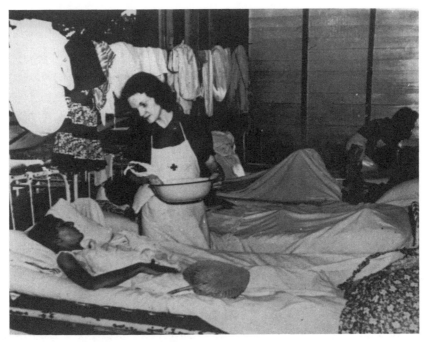

A Japanese guard took this photograph of Peg at Santo Tomas for propaganda purposes. The photo circulated all the way to her hometown of Wilkes-Barre, Pennsylvania. *Courtesy of Bureau of Medicine and Surgery*

treated. The photograph spread all the way to her hometown in Pennsylvania, where her mother confirmed that yes, it was her Peggy.

Peg's mother and the other nurses' families were unsure what to think. The newspapers wrongly reported how the Santo Tomas inmates had "the run of the old University grounds" and were permitted to take language classes and other stimulating courses. The diet, supplied by the Philippine Red Cross, included vegetables and meat. Inmates' health was described as "good" and morale as "excellent." The experience sounded a bit like summer camp.

But the propaganda material distributed by the US War Department painted a more realistic portrait. One illustration depicted six beautiful young nurses, wearing crisp white uniforms, navy blue capes, and mournful expressions. They stood trapped behind barbed wire, guarded by a grotesque Japanese soldier. At the same time, the US Army capitalized on the breathtaking testimonies of nurses who had escaped from Corregidor. Army nurse Juanita Redmond survived the bombing at Hospital #1 and published a memoir in early 1943 about her experiences in Bataan. She also awkwardly delivered lines for a propaganda film and spoke at war bond drives. Other liberated or evacuated nurses from Guam and the Philippines also gave lectures nationwide. After their compelling talks, the women implored audiences to support the war effort and help liberate the captive nurses.

Behind the barbed wire at Los Baños, the men arrived, parched and pained. They expected the guards to assign dormitories, or at least allow the newly elected administrative committee* to divvy up sleeping arrangements. But the guards had no intention of distributing food, water, or mosquito nets. The entire camp was ordered to the baseball diamond. Dorothy huddled on the turf with the other nurses, swatting at the mosquitos and sharing whatever scraps of food they had brought with them or a kind Filipino had hurled into the passing boxcar as they rolled past. As the sun set and darkness bled through the sky, the inmates realized they were being held indefinitely. Angry voices hissed reminders that the Geneva Convention forbade exposing prisoners to the elements. The guards were unmoved.

Dorothy leaned back and looked the sky. Starlight bit through the blackness, and visible constellations appeared. After years of living in Manila, she was finally able to see all the stars obscured by the city lights. Under the expansive night sky, it was easy for an inmate to remember how minute she was in the vast universe. Perhaps this was what the guards intended when they forced the camp out onto

---

* The Santo Tomas inmates labeled their leadership as the "executive committee." At Los Baños, they used the term "administrative committee," intending for the administrative group to report to the executive committee after the two camps fully merged.

the baseball diamond—to provoke a sense of insignificance in a big world, and prompt the inmates to wonder whether anyone outside the Philippines ever thought about them at all.

At dawn, the inmates picked at the raised welts that spotted their bodies. Mosquitos had feasted during the night and added to their misery. At least, Dorothy thought, they were in the mountains, and unlikely to contract malaria after their night of forced exposure.

The baseball diamond emptied as inmates eagerly claimed their small pocket of the prison. The administrative committee had arranged for the men to occupy a large gymnasium until barracks were constructed. The nurses were given their own dormitory. After sharing a classroom with more than fifty other inmates, the nurses were divided into small rooms of three women each. It practically felt private.

The nurses had another sliver of good fortune that afternoon. Near the barbed wire fence, the women noticed a small flock of chickens that had mistakenly wandered into the camp. The women quietly discussed a strategy for catching a bird. Basilia Torres Steward offered to kill, pluck, and cook the whole chicken if only they could snag one of them. A chicken stew, she suggested, would make the most of the meat. The nurses obsessed over the idea but talked themselves out of it. Then they reconsidered, tempted by the possibility of stew for dinner.

The chicken was indeed high-risk, high-reward. The guards at Santa Tomas typically ignored the inmates unless they ventured toward the perimeter. The women had to assume the Los Baños guards would shoot to kill if they mistook the chicken chase for an attempted escape. The nurses decided only one of them would try for the capture while the rest focused their attention on the guard, prepared to intervene with some sort of distraction if he noticed one of the women nearing the forbidden fence.

Petite, sweet Eldene Paige, the nurse who wrote poetry to console herself, surprised everyone by volunteering to run the mission. She had experience with chickens, having been born in South Dakota and raised on a farm in Southern California. She knew how to walk among a flock without causing a disruption. Eldene crept toward the barbed wire. She saw that one of the birds was injured and immobile. She slunk like a fox toward the flock and swiftly pounced on the debilitated bird.

The nurses watched with delight as Eldene carried the struggling creature toward them. Basilia expertly grabbed the bird by the feet, pulled down on the neck and twisted forcefully. She lowered the bird into boiling water to loosen the feathers. Almost every part of the chicken had value to the women. The feathers could be stuffed into a pillow or mattress. The bones could be boiled multiple times to create a broth. And the gizzards could be fried and served over rice. The rest of the inmates had only canned rations—corned beef and hard crackers—to look forward to after a long day of setting up camp. The women each enjoyed a warm bowl of chicken stew.

The nurses reported to the infirmary the next morning. Dorothy was relieved to find that it was a proper clinic. At Santo Tomas they had started the hospital in an old machine shop and then set up wards in various buildings, including the old convent. Their new infirmary had an actual waiting room, beyond which was a hallway lined with doors opening into several wards as well as a surgical suite. A wrought-iron stairwell twisted down to the basement, where there was a pharmacy, storage, a kitchen to prepare patient meals, and living quarters.

The nurses explored the infirmary, wandering through open doors and looking for where the medical equipment was stashed. The rooms were completely empty, and the nurses' movements sent echoes around the bare walls. American and Filipino troops had previously occupied the university and stripped it of valuables before evacuating. Occupying forces moving through the area had done more of the same.

Dorothy found the surgical suite and the remnants left after it was ransacked. Little remained except an antiquated washbowl and surgical table that were bolted to the floor. She walked over to an instrument sterilizer and peered inside. She saw specks of rice dotting the sides, an indication that someone had once tried to use it to boil water for rice. The sterilizer was dead from abuse.

In the wards, the nurses looked at each other with disbelief. There was nothing left, and they had brought almost no supplies from Santo Tomas—the camp commanders had forcefully restricted what the nurses could take with them. They had nothing to work with. No bandages or sutures, tongue depressors, or adhesives. No plaster of paris to make casts or slings to support healing limbs. No medicine. The women didn't even have glasses in which to offer a patient a drink of water. And where would a patient rest? There were no beds or linens. Even the cabinets had been ripped from the walls.

The first few patients in the infirmary brought their own bed-rolls. In the coming weeks, innovative inmates would use pipes to fit together bedsteads. They pried open seed pods from nearby bulak trees and plucked the soft cotton-like fluff to stuff into mattresses and pillows. The mattresses were then covered with jusi, a sheer type of fabric woven from the stringy fibers found inside banana leaves. The threadlike strings were also woven into mosquito nets and strung over patient beds. For call bells, the nurses hung a mobile of empty beer bottles a patient could clatter to signal when assistance was needed.

As self-reliant survivors of the Great Depression, the women possessed skills such as sewing and gardening. Surgical nurse Goldia O'Haver was an exceptional seamstress. She sat down at an antiquated sewing machine and turned heaps of unbleached muslin into sheets.

Inmates donated old clothes and fabric scraps for Goldia to make pillowcases, surgical gowns, and patient pajamas. Goldia also secured a bolt of blue denim, which she used to make uniforms for the nurses. In exchange for receiving two new uniforms each, the nurses turned over their old despised dungarees and impractical white uniforms. Goldia repurposed the uniforms as bandages.

Repurposing was key, and ingenuity was crucial in a poorly stocked pharmacy. The nurses treated coughs with a mixture of sugar and onion juice, and prescribed guava leaf tea for bacillary dysentery. On the advice of locals, the women also experimented with mango leaf to treat diabetes, but they found it did not effectively lower blood sugar as promised. The nurses had more success with the bandage adhesive supplied by several inmates who had been pharmaceutical

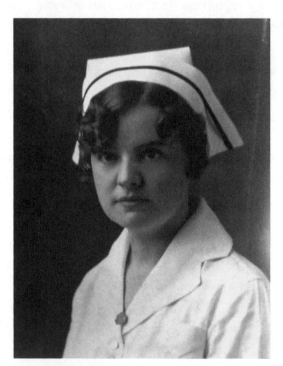

Navy nurse Goldia O'Haver. *Courtesy of Bureau of Medicine and Surgery*

representatives before the war. The pharmacy men tapped a nearby rubber tree and mixed the sap with various bases, experimenting until the right concoction developed.

In the coming months, the infirmary began to resemble the hospital the nurses envisioned. Inmates with woodworking skills made new cabinets as well as dressing tables. They also whittled bamboo into tongue depressors and applicator sticks. They ripped up wild-growing reed and cut the tall grass into drinking straws. Meanwhile, the camp electricians rewired the instrument sterilizer and engineered a bicycle-powered battery charger. And volunteers sawed and smoothed tin cans into drinking cups.

Medical supplies trickled into the infirmary, mostly as a result of firm negotiations with a hapless Japanese medical sergeant. The sergeant was responsible for the seventy-five-man garrison and he was overwhelmed by their questions and concerns. The sergeant sought daily advice from the nurses and often asked the physician to look at dysentery slides. The women were tight lipped unless the sergeant had something to offer. If he wanted medical advice, then he had to pay through sutures, bandages, or drugs like insulin for the diabetics and antibacterial treatments for patients with jungle rot. The latter condition was a particular scourge in the early months, as the tropical climate and unsanitary conditions turned inmates' flesh into open wounds. Lines of men waited to sit with their infected feet in a tub filled with bichloride of mercury, a compound once used to treat the open sores caused by syphilis.

The camp commander admired how quickly the inmates organized the camp. The work gave inmates something productive to do, which helped alleviate the oppressive boredom of imprisonment. But the commander was misguided if he thought the inmates were cheerful worker bees. This wasn't *Swiss Family Robinson*, and none of them took delight in having to repurpose or reinvent basic necessities. Several inmates, however, did find pleasure in building clandestine radios and listening to news about the war. Gerald Sams, the former radio operator at Cavite, took particular enjoyment every time a guard searched his quarters and unwittingly glanced over the sewing supply box that concealed his secret radio. At times, Gerald even pointed out the wooden box and boasted how he had made it himself, hoping to elicit compliments on the craftsmanship.

The guards also noted the nurses' resourcefulness and even tried to use it to their own advantage. A sentry once interrupted Mary Rose and Basilia in the infirmary. He did not speak English or Tagalog, but he tried to pantomime a mending request as he held out a pair of pants he wished to have stitched. Basilia's eyes widened at the request. She'd lost everything in her life to the Japanese army. Her husband was in a prison camp, and she had been separated from her family, ostensibly for her own protection. Every personal item she owned fit into a small trunk. And the majority of her time outside of the infirmary was devoted to extending the lifespan of her dwindling personal effects. *String* was a valuable possession, and this guard wanted his pants stitched?

Basilia refused. "Take them outside," she said. "A Filipino will do them."

Because she knew he didn't understand her words, Basilia lowered her head in the Filipino manner of saying "No." She pointed at the door to indicate that the sentry would not find a seamstress within the camp. The sentry acquiesced. He tucked the pants beneath his arm and left the infirmary quietly. Feigned deference had its limits.

———————

Just as the infirmary was coming together, the commanders pulled it apart. In August, about two dozen inmates were plucked from Los Baños to be repatriated in a prisoner exchange. Dr. Leach, the prison's only physician, somehow made the cut, which the nurses surmised was due to his employment by the Rockefeller Foundation. The medical team was now limited to the twelve nurses, a dentist, a few pharmaceutical representatives, and a PhD who focused his attention on the sanitation system. For a month, the nurses managed on their own. They knew how to handle the ailments that patients presented. But they still needed a surgeon.

In mid-September, Dr. Dana Nance transferred from another camp. The nurses quickly learned that Dana was a man with his own rule book. At age thirty-eight, he had no military background; he was born in Tennessee but raised primarily in Asia by his missionary parents. He had returned to the United States long enough to attend medical school and meet and marry his dimple-cheeked wife, Anna. The couple relocated to Shanghai and had three children. Dana sent his family back to America when the State Department began issuing warnings about China. He then relocated to the Philippines, assuming it was safe because it was under American protection. He was taken prisoner after the invasion and sent to Baguio prison camp, about 150 miles north of Manila.

The nurses were excited that Dana had brought surgical instruments, but they did not have a good first impression of the doctor himself. Soon after Dana arrived, the medical sergeant for the Japanese garrison came to the infirmary with a grave concern. A civilian working for the commander was complaining of severe abdominal pain. Dana agreed to examine the patient and found the civilian's appendix close to bursting. The commander wanted to transfer the civilian to Manila for surgery, but Dana argued that the man would not survive the trip. He urged the commander to allow him to operate.

The women were not keen on the idea. Dana persisted, and the commander retreated to his office to consider his options. The civilian was one of the commander's favorites. After hours of deliberation, the commander told Dana to move forward with the surgery. But his permission came with one condition. If the man died on the table, one of the nurses would be shot in retaliation. The nurses resented the renegade physician who had now put one of their lives on the line.

The patient was brought into the surgery that evening, guarded by a soldier with his bayonet drawn. Nurse anesthetist Susie Pitcher took her place near the operating table. Goldia scrubbed in and stood ready to assist. Mary Rose was assigned the task of circulating in the surgery, bringing sterilized instruments or whatever the surgeon requested. And Chief Nurse Cobb invited herself into the room, feeling instinctively responsible for her nurses.

Susie picked up the ether can and masterfully applied the right dose to a gauze mask. The mask was placed over the patient's nose and mouth, and his eyelids became heavy as he breathed in the anesthetic. Goldia passed Dana a scalpel and watched as he made an incision on the patient's lower abdomen. She handed the surgeon a pair of scissors to widen the cut and then pinched one side of the incision open as Dana worked to cut through tissue and muscle. Susie monitored the patient's breathing, ready to respond if he showed signs of consciousness.

The nurses tensely watched as Dana pulled the appendix through the incision. It was indeed as inflamed as he expected. Mary Rose brought the surgeon a suture, and he tied up the end of the appendix to prevent the deadly bacteria from seeping back into the body. Dana trimmed the thread and snipped the appendix, and Goldia quickly blotted the blood from the large intestine while Dana inspected his suture. Satisfied, he tucked the intestine back into the abdomen. Goldia held the incision open as Dana threaded the layers of tissue and muscle. After he sewed the skin closed, Goldia cleaned off the blood and one of the nurses, likely Mary Rose, applied antiseptic to the wound. The patient was transferred to the ward for recovery. The nurses were relieved as he surfaced into consciousness. The ordeal was over.

The nurses then stepped into the moonlit evening. The bright moonlight reminded Mary Rose of another evening, when she'd come upon a guard staring dreamily at a full moon. "I'm homesick," he announced, as if his problems might interest her.

But the guards' problems did not interest the inmates. And now they were angry with Dana for making a Japanese civilian's problem their problem, risking one of their lives in the process. If Dana hoped to be well liked at Los Baños, he would first have to redeem himself with the twelve nurses. He was an unknown surgeon new to a population of inmates who had suffered together for almost two years. He would eventually learn that the nurses were the camp's anchors. And although they needed him, Dana needed the twelve anchors even more.

11

I Am Ashamed of You

DOROTHY DUG THROUGH her footlocker. She did not open the trunk often, because it contained reminders of her life before the war. Such memories, she thought, had the potential to make her cry. But today was special, and she wanted to look her best. She sorted through the civilian attire she'd previously worn to dinners and dances. She rummaged past the dry-clean-only dresses and considered donating them to the infirmary. Edwina could make use of them for arm slings, surgical robes, or patient pajamas.

Dorothy pulled out a pressed dress and held it up. It had been years since she'd dressed up. She collected her small cosmetics jars, dabbed makeup on her face, and smoothed her freshly rinsed hair. She left the nurses' quarters and walked to the makeshift classroom where she was scheduled to teach an introductory course to men who had volunteered as orderlies. Dorothy knew the orderlies would never reach the same level as her corpsmen, but the nurses needed extra hands in the infirmary. All twenty-five beds in the ward were filled, and the clinic Peg ran for outpatient treatment was in steady demand. On a typical day, Peg had at least fifteen men sitting with their feet in a medicated tub, trying to alleviate the oozing sores caused by jungle rot. During the rainy season, Peg also saw an increase in broken bones or sprained ligaments among prisoners navigating the slick mud that coated the camp.

The infirmary was understaffed, and the nurses worried how they would manage after more inmates were transferred in from Santo Tomas. Dorothy approached Chief Nurse Cobb with the idea of an orderly training program. Cobb liked the suggestion but felt the potential candidates would need review. There were too many men in the camp who were anxious for female company and likely to apply in hopes of winning one of the nurses as a girlfriend. There were also some men who lacked the physical strength or mental aptitude. After all candidates were considered, twelve men were selected for the first class of orderly trainees.

Mary Rose agreed to help Dorothy with the training and provided her with a copy of the Navy Hospital Corps handbook. The weighty book was nearly one thousand pages long, and Dorothy mulled over the text for weeks, trying to decide how to introduce basic nursing concepts to men without a medical background. She was often sidetracked by reading the handbook's regulations for handling food and supplies, which she hadn't seen in years. The kitchen refrigerator, for example, was supposed to be restocked each evening with eggs, fruit, and milk. Dietitian Bertha Evans hadn't been able to properly stock a fridge since their time at Cavite. Similarly, the sections on cleaning were almost painful to read. The handbook included a small passage on practicing self-care, which stipulated proper water intake, dietary habits, and daily bathing as a fundamental requirement of the job. The last time Dorothy received a bar of soap was in the January comfort kit. She lathered with the little bar until only a sliver remained, which she then saved in her trunk, if only to count it among her paltry possessions.

The handbook made Dorothy reflect on who she had been before the war, and who she had become as her time in captivity degraded her. On the first day of the class, she wanted to look as presentable as she could, wearing civilian dress. All eyes were on Dorothy as she walked into the room and began arranging the instruments she planned to demonstrate. She paused and looked up at the dozens of men watching her set up. She had expected only the twelve selected men to attend the training, yet there was a crowd of unfamiliar faces. She knew these men had not received acceptance to train, and she thought they were confused about the purpose of the meeting. Internees regularly hosted language courses or history lectures, and she assumed there was a scheduling error.

"This is a class for the hospital orderlies," she explained.

Dorothy expected the interlopers to realize their mistake and leave the room. Instead, the men smiled back at her. They looked her up and down, admired her figure and her blond hair. A few, hoping to engage her in conversation, admitted they hadn't been accepted as orderlies but were considering putting in a future application, perhaps when the other prisoners transferred from Santo Tomas. Until then, they just wanted to watch her class.

Dorothy backed out the door. "Gentlemen, please don't go away," she called to the room. She hustled to her dormitory and changed out of her dress. She pulled on her blue denim uniform, which modestly hung past her knees and blurred her figure. Giant buttons ran from the chest to the skirt, and gave the woman wearing it the appearance of a schoolmarm. Dorothy hurried back to the makeshift classroom and reassumed her position at the front. Her admirers sensed her seriousness and slunk from the room.

At the time, Dorothy thought the men who came to gaze at her were just missing their wives and sweethearts and wanted a small reminder of their home life. She tended to disregard the fact that she was a beautiful young woman whom men saw as desirable. Dorothy had a similar naïveté regarding a charming inmate who actively pursued her attention.

Thomas S. Terrill, who had grown up in Southern California, was a year older than Dorothy. He joined the military with the goal of becoming a pilot. His service separated him from his girlfriend, Margaret, a comely brunette from Pasadena. But before his commitment was complete, Margaret traveled to Texas and married him near base. After his discharge, Thomas flew for the Consolidated Aircraft Company of San Diego and the couple moved to New York City. Their early years of marriage were probably lonely for Margaret, who was far from home in New York while Thomas piloted routes to the Caribbean and Central America. He was gone for lengthy stretches, leaving Margaret and their young son alone in a strange city.

Consolidated Aircraft sent Thomas to Manila in November 1941, just weeks before Pearl Harbor was bombed. After the attack, he secured a seat on a flight home but was bumped by men with more seniority. The missed flight was his one opportunity to evacuate, and in January 1942, Thomas was ordered to report to Santo Tomas as a civilian internee. He'd had few opportunities to communicate with Margaret in the past years. On several occasions, the various commanders at Santo Tomas allowed the Red Cross to distribute preprinted postcards in which inmates answered questions such as "My health is . . ." by circling benign options of good, fair, or poor. He knew Margaret had brought their young family back to Southern California and given birth to their second son, whom he had yet to meet.

Dorothy first met Thomas while relaxing on the lawn one evening with several other nurses. He introduced himself as a fellow Southern Californian and sat alongside her. Thomas was a handsome man, with light brown hair and full lips. He approached Dorothy as a friend, claiming to only have the intention of reminiscing about his life before the war. Their early conversations revolved around the fact that they had once lived close to each other in Long Beach. They named various restaurants and playgrounds they had frequented as children and joked they had probably destroyed each other's sand castles at the beach.

Dorothy avoided admitting that Thomas had a romantic interest in her. She rationalized that he just wanted to be reminded of his home. But Thomas was a graduate of Cal Tech, located in nurse Edwina's hometown. Thomas didn't pursue Edwina to talk about Pasadena, or how she had attended the same junior college as his wife. Edwina actually graduated from the nursing program the same year his wife attended as an English major. Yet Thomas didn't register the connection. Nor did he try to engage nurse Eldene in conversations about the years she lived in Long Beach and Lomita. Thomas wasn't seeking a connection to Southern California, he was seeking a relationship with Dorothy.

Dorothy liked Thomas's attention and allowed time to visit with him daily. Their hours together often came at the end of the evening after the stars were out. They would find a quiet spot on the baseball diamond or soccer field away from the other inmates, where they could stretch back and look at the web of constellations. Thomas had long appreciated astronomy, and he named the constellations and pointed out planets. Dorothy looked at the sky and back at the smiling man next to her. She tried to stop herself from falling in love, but life at home seemed a forgotten memory. The lives they endured in the camp, with their slivers of soap and tin can drinking cups, bore no resemblance to their past. Their loved ones at home couldn't help them here in Los Baños. The only people who mattered were their allies in the camp.

Other bonds were also forming among the nurses. A man with impressive carpentry skills admired nurse Peg. Upon her request, he worked on the nurses' quarters and added wooden floors and cup-boards. He also helped with construction projects around the infir-mary, such as building cabinets and a dressing cart. The women teased Peg, noting that she only had to suggest to her friend, *"Wouldn't it be nice if..."* and then work would promptly begin. Goldia O'Haver attracted the interest of Robert Merrill, an army mechanic from New Hampshire. Even Chief Nurse Cobb had a friend, Hugh Williams, a retired naval captain from New Zealand, whose cheerful disposition, Dorothy thought, contrasted with Cobb's brusque manner.

Mary Rose also fell in love. Her beau, T. Page Nelson, worked for the Treasury Department. He had transferred to Manila in the summer of 1941 to freeze Japanese assets. Like so many other civil-ians, he was unable to evacuate and reported to Santo Tomas with the understanding that the internment was a mere registration pro-cess and he would be released within days. Now, almost twenty months later, he tried to make the best of his imprisonment by serving on committees and participating in athletic events. He signed up for a track meet one day but injured his ankle during practice. He limped to the infirmary, where the auburn-haired Mary Rose was on duty. Page was immediately smitten. He was determined to hover near his nurse. The camp had several hundred bachelors vying for female attention. Page applied to Dorothy's orderly program. He also rounded up a few friends, cleaned out an unoccupied area of the infirmary basement, and moved into the room. Anytime he wasn't working or sleeping, Page found himself an excuse to be near Mary Rose.

Thomas Terrill also sought reasons to visit Dorothy, but there was a clear distinction between the two pairs. Page was twenty-three and a single man. He and Mary Rose openly spoke of marriage and building a life together after the war. Thomas, Dorothy knew, planned to return to his wife after liberation. At times, the thought of losing Thomas was so painful that Dorothy tried to distance herself. Thomas

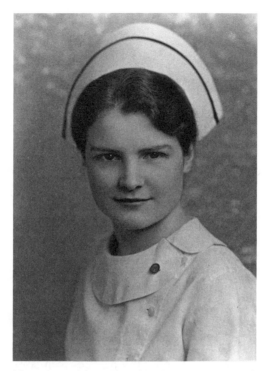

Navy nurse Mary Rose Harrington. *Courtesy of Bureau of Medicine and Surgery*

always found a way to bring her back to him. Even if the relationship was unsustainable, it was undeniable, and it came at a time when Dorothy needed a friend.

———————

Tensions were increasing at the hospital. The nurses were still adjusting to the new surgeon, as well as the well-meaning but unskilled orderlies. The nurses were glad to have help lifting patients or emptying bedpans, but they were critical when the orderlies made mistakes. A few of the women recalled their own fumbling days as probationary nurses and tried to avoid humiliating the men. But others were open with their criticism and blamed Dorothy for doing a poor job of training the help. Friction arose between Dorothy and Helen after an inept orderly treated a scabies patient with the wrong solution. The patient had small raised welts caused by mites burrowing into his skin and laying eggs. The nurses typically remedied scabies with gentian violet, but the orderly instead grabbed an iodine bottle and painted the patient's skin with a thick smear. The already irritated skin burned from the iodine, and Helen confronted Dorothy.

Dorothy stiffened when Helen reported how one of her "stupid corpsmen" had confused the two medicines. These men were not her corpsmen. Her *actual* corpsmen were not properly regarded as noncombatants and Dorothy had heard they were suffering in the military camps. Had Helen forgotten? Had she failed to remember they were in a prison? Helen corrected herself: OK, one of Dorothy's "stupid orderlies" had burned a patient. "It was your idea to teach them," she scowled.

Helen unkindly told Dorothy how she should teach the orderlies. Dorothy had no interest in receiving advice from someone who had grumbled when they lacked help and now complained about the quality of the help. "Oh, stick it in your ear!" Dorothy hissed.

Chief Nurse Cobb overheard the commotion. "Miss Still!" she scolded from the doorway.

Cobb paused and considered the situation. She did not have all the details of the dispute, but she did know one of her nurses had just told another where to shove it. She focused her attention on Dorothy. "Must I remind you that you are in the Navy Nurse Corps?"

Dorothy nodded obediently as Cobb sniffed at her "unladylike behavior." The two angry nurses walked away from the conflict, each one feeling it was not yet over.

Within a few days, they picked up the same fight after one of the orderlies allowed a dysentery patient to eat a papaya. Dysentery was deadly in the prison camps. The highly contagious bacteria spread through contaminated food, water, or hand-to-mouth contact. The bacteria infected the intestines and caused bloody diarrhea and high fever. Weakened and abused prisoners were unable to survive it. At Los Baños, dysentery patients had been given a strict diet, which excluded aggravating fruits such as papaya.

Helen was furious with the mistake. She confronted Dorothy at the infirmary's front desk. Helen listed all the problems she felt the orderlies were causing, and Dorothy fired back with the suggestion that Helen should train the men herself if she thought she could do a better job. Their angry voices blasted through the walls as they accused each other of being defensive. The patients within the wards perked up with the entertaining sounds of unfolding drama. In the basement, Cobb heard the commotion and ran up the stairs toward the shouting.

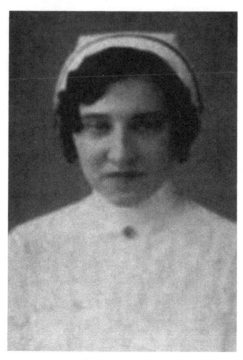

Navy nurse Helen C. Gorzelanski. *Courtesy of Bureau of Medicine and Surgery*

Both women went silent as they saw Cobb hustling down the hallway. "Ladies!" she demanded. "What is this about?"

Helen shrugged. Dorothy attempted to deny there was a problem. Cobb ordered the women to keep their arguments out of the infirmary. Then she passed a hard and fast judgment as to who was at fault for the situation. "Miss Still," she scolded. "I am ashamed of you."

"Yes, ma'am," Dorothy acknowledged.

Dorothy skulked away from the front desk feeling waves of resentment and humiliation. In the ward, she forged a smile and tried to pretend she'd had nothing to do with the yelling match that everyone in the hospital had heard word for word. Her shift was nearly over, and she made her final rounds and focused on finishing her reports. Before she left, she went to the front desk to give Helen her shift reports. Helen felt the argument was not finished, and she chided Dorothy's "juvenile behavior." Dorothy considered giving Helen a sentry-style crack across the cheek. She stormed out the front door instead.

Thomas lurked in the area as he tended to do toward the end of Dorothy's shift. He heard the infirmary door slam angrily behind her and caught up as she stomped down the road. Dorothy barely acknowledged Thomas as he walked alongside her. In her mind, she envisioned Chief Nurse Cobb taking out the nurses' records—the same ones she had hidden during transport—and making a permanent note of Dorothy's conduct. The reprimand burned Dorothy. She wasn't even supposed to be there! Her orders had been to leave the Philippines on January 1, 1942. Instead, the navy forgot about the nurses. Almost two years later, she still maintained her position even though no one was requiring her to, and now the thanks she got from her chief nurse was a critical note on her record?

"Want to talk about it?" Thomas asked.

Dorothy let all her anger spill out. She told Thomas the full story, and realized it was a conflict she would have handled much differently in peacetime. The women were simply exhausted. They had been making do with so little for so long. Frustration weighed on them, and every day was a reminder of the life and the people they had lost. The orderlies, as needed as they were in the infirmary, were also a reminder of the corpsmen who the nurses knew were suffering gravely. Couriers continued to ferry secret notes between the military and civilian prison camps. Forced work crews from both prisons still met at the Manila pier and whispered messages. And the shuttle bus that ran from Santo Tomas to Los Baños relayed the bad news—their corpsmen were dying in hell, and there was nothing the nurses could do to stop their pain.

Dorothy seemed to recognize that Helen had the same frustrations and fears. The two women never spoke of the incident again, and instead quietly forgave each other. Several days later, Helen approached Dorothy with a pair of scissors and asked for a haircut. Dorothy, with her steady hand, was the resident stylist. Helen sat in front of Dorothy as she gently combed and trimmed her hair into a chin-length cut. It was a style popular in Hollywood before the war, which in some ways was where the inmates still resided. They were essentially frozen in December 1941, when they were ripped from their lives and trapped in a time loop. The rest of the world moved forward, but they cycled through the same misery month after month.

———————

Dorothy sat on the examination table as Dana Nance and Chief Nurse Cobb came into the room. Obediently, she lay back and allowed her skirt to be raised as Dana examined the swollen mound that distended near her pubic area. The doctor diagnosed the bulge as a hernia. He thought a loop of her intestines had pushed through a weak spot in her abdominal wall. He wanted to operate immediately—hernias could be deadly if the tear in the abdominal wall tightened around the intestine and constricted the oxygen supply.

Dorothy thought she had likely developed the hernia by lifting a patient or heavy object such as a bed. But she hesitated to have surgery as Dana suggested. She suspected he just had the itch to operate, and she wanted to wait to see if the injury would heal on its own. Cobb encouraged Dorothy to undergo the procedure, agreeing with the doctor that her condition could bring severe complications if left untreated. And the chief nurse could not guarantee how long they would have the anesthesia necessary to painlessly perform such surgeries. Now was the time, she urged.

Dorothy soon found herself on the operating table, watching as nurse anesthetist Susie Pitcher lowered a gauze mask to her nose. Dorothy smelled the sweetness of the ether as the figures in front of her blurred into a haze. She blinked her eyes closed and then reopened them in the recovery room. Her surgery, she learned, was indeed lifesaving. The hernia had caused a hydrocele, which was a pooling of fluid. While Dana repaired the hernia and drained the fluid, he sensed the need to also examine her appendix. He tugged the appendix through the incision and saw that it was inflamed and ready to burst.

Dorothy was initially stunned at how close she had come to death. Early in her captivity, she'd made her peace with the prospect of dying young. In her contemplations, she assumed the possibilities of dying in the internment camp ranged from violence to starvation to infectious disease. An appendix removal was a commonplace emergency that even schoolchildren experienced. It was odd for Dorothy to think her parents might have received a telegram reporting her death—not from a tropical disease or a guard's bullet but from a burst appendix.

Dorothy's thoughts about her own mortality were soon replaced with boredom. Her incision was healing and the pain was subsiding. She felt ready to return to work, a request that Cobb promptly refused. Postsurgical hernia patients had to convalesce for three weeks.

Dorothy felt useless lying in bed, particularly because both Basilia and Cobb were also ill and the infirmary was understaffed.

While she recovered, the other nurses brought Dorothy the materials she needed to help make Christmas gifts for the children at Santo Tomas. Both camps were again turning their attention to the holiday season as a distraction, and one of the Christmas committees had requested two hundred toys. The prisoners in Dorothy's camp were preoccupied with rebuilding after a violent typhoon swept through the Philippines. The barracks' thatched roofs had collapsed from the weight of water, and the inmates hurriedly rebuilt their shelters. Toy making was not high on the priority list, but Dorothy gladly accepted the task.

Dorothy hoped the Christmas gifts would help rebuild morale in Santo Tomas. Covert communication revealed that the camp was becoming increasingly diseased and violent. The population soared to thirty-nine hundred people, and with food shortages, the restaurant served only two meals a day. Breakfast was gruel, which the inmates said looked and tasted like wallpaper paste. Dinner was a scant mixture of vegetables and the occasional duck egg. Inmates with money could no longer buy their way out of starvation. The Japanese-run canteen was out of sugar, lard, and rice. At the infirmary, patients presented with symptoms of malnutrition and the medical staff was helpless to respond. The depleted infirmary lacked even basic supplies such as iodine and disinfectants.

The shortages at Santo Tomas were intentional. The camp's warrant officer slashed rations to heighten suffering, and he intended to use his power to convert Santo Tomas from a prison camp into a slow-motion death camp. The process was interrupted when his commander allowed the Red Cross to distribute comfort kits in mid-December. The comfort kits briefly raised inmates' daily nutrition, but it also depleted their morale. It was the scenario that Colorado native Abraham Hartendorp had envisioned the year before when he saw desperate inmates squeezing margarine into their mouths. The promise of comfort kits had the ability to emotionally wreck the inmates.

With the new delivery, the sentries claimed patriotic messages were hidden in the wrappers of the Old Gold cigarettes. Indeed, the tobacco company had printed a promise to fight for the American way of life: "Our heritage has always been freedom—We cannot afford to relinquish it—Our armed forces will safeguard that heritage if we do our share to preserve it."

The guards responded by ransacking the kits looking for covert communications. A hungry crowd formed to watch the sentries rip through the packages. The guards sliced open tins and poured the contents on the ground. Cans of corn beef and salmon were punctured, opened, and discarded. Mothers wailed as cans of condensed milk were dumped in front of their children. News of the desecration ripped through the camp, and other inmates abandoned their work details and ran toward the hysterical crowd.

The guards tired of the search after destroying several hundred kits. Members of the executive committee promptly confronted the commander, and arrangements were made to begin distribution that afternoon to children and teenagers. The rest of the camp had to wait for their kits while all contents were searched. The ugly behavior that had come with the previous comfort kits was repeated, this time with the children first. One boy was hospitalized after he ate an entire high-calorie chocolate bar intended to be consumed at a rate of one square per day. And a three-year-old girl walked through the camp, showing off a wedge of cheese and bag of prunes and boasting to hungry adults that she had more back in her shanty.

The commander regarded the comfort kits as though they were an extravagant gift the ragged inmates did not deserve. There had to be limits on privileges, and although the commander allowed inmates to receive gift baskets on Christmas Day, he forbade the family visits he had permitted the previous year. Weeping spouses pleaded at the gate for entry and then left in defeat. A gloom settled over the camp, and the holidays were notably subdued. Although the programming and homemade gifts had provided a distraction, the inmates seemed glad when the festivities were over.

At Los Baños, Christmas was also restrained but still a welcome diversion. A choir prepared a performance of Christmas carols and the drama society decided to replicate the play *The Philadelphia Story* as a radio broadcast performed over the loudspeaker. The story was an outlandish tale about a handsome reporter investigating a Philadelphia socialite as she tries to remarry for status. Nurse Peg had a role in the performance, which preoccupied her as she recovered in the hospital from dengue fever.

Peg shared a hospital room with Dorothy. She practiced her lines and distracted herself with worry the drama society would give the role to someone else if she was unable to recover. The diversion had its limits, and Peg nursed deep anxiety about her ability to survive the war. She revealed her concerns to Dorothy, whispering across the small room that she didn't want to die in the Philippines. If she were to die young, she wanted to be buried with her family in Pennsylvania. She grimaced at the thought of being pushed under the mud at Los Baños.

"You can't die here," Dorothy agreed. "You don't have a decent thing to be buried in."

Part IV

1944

———

12

We Might Not Come Out of This Alive

THE INMATES AT Santo Tomas internment camp were hungry and humiliated. Yet for all their hardships, they suspected they were experiencing better conditions than the other civilian or military camps. The military men at Bilibid Prison continued to send forbidden notes smuggled through couriers. The messages begged for supplies and revealed that countless inmates had died from disease, neglect, and violence. At Cabanatuan, the military camp north of Manila, the prisoners wrote about forced farm labor and daily beatings. There were multiple instances in which men were forced to dig their own graves.

The Santo Tomas inmates also did not envy the prisoners who had left for Los Baños. As expected, the commander's promise of a health resort had never materialized. Nor had a sewage system. The new camp's water supply tested positive for *E. coli*, and inmates were directed to boil their drinking water. The task proved too cumbersome, and the inmates took to sipping straight from the spigot. The most nauseating stories to seep back from Los Baños, however, referenced the bathrooms. Without running water, the inmates had to improvise a flush system. The "toilets" consisted of a cement trough with a panel of wood laid atop it; six cutouts in the wood were covered neatly with toilet seats. The trough sloped slightly down toward a septic tank. On the higher end, a water closet intermittently released a stream to flush the contents toward the tank. Back at Santo Tomas, the inmates figured they had to wait in long lines to use the toilets but at least they had running water and electricity. Los Baños seemed like a step down, and many inmates refused to consider a transfer, even as more prisoners were crammed into Santo Tomas.

To add to the overcrowding, five busloads of inmates from the Davao prison camp on the southern island of Mindanao arrived at Santo Tomas in early January. Inmates gathered near the main building to watch the newcomers unload. They were stunned by the Davao inmates' ragged appearance. The men, women, and children were flea-bitten and emaciated. They looked exhausted and filthy after spending more than a week on a slow-moving ship to Manila. The new arrivals stumbled from the buses and trudged into a registration line that fed into the commander's office. A redheaded woman stood among the crowd, hoping to see her family among the newcomers. Days before Pearl Harbor, the woman had traveled from the southern Philippine island to Manila to shop for Christmas presents for her husband and children—a four-year-old daughter, two-year-old son, and baby boy. She was stranded in Manila after the Japanese attacked and had been forced into internment at Santo Tomas.

Twenty-five months had passed since she'd seen her loved ones. She scanned the crowd, looking for her children's distinct red hair. The registration process took hours, and she stared intently at the new arrivals, searching for recognition in the unfamiliar faces. She had no assurance that her family was among the transfers, or if they were even still alive. And then she saw them emerge from the main building. She released a hysterical scream and ducked under the partition.

The crowd watched as she raced to her daughter and pulled her into a tight embrace. She gripped her older son next, and he flinched in fear at the strange woman trying to grab him. She crouched alongside her toddler and tugged off his cap. She stroked his red locks, amazed at the small child her little baby had become. The woman cried as she hugged her children, partly out of relief, but also with complete devastation. Her sons did not recognize her.

The reunion released other inmates' emotions, and bystanders dabbed tears from their own cheeks. They understood why the children did not recognize a woman they hadn't seen in two years. In the camps, it was the people who stood alongside an inmate who mattered most, not the family members who could not help. Distant family was like a faint, glowing light—a reason to continue living. But fellow inmates were the ones who kept a prisoner alive.

That was the peculiarity of Santo Tomas. On the surface, it seemed to be much better than the other camps. But the layers of misery ran deep. Spouses were separated from each other, and children were ripped from their parents. Many in the camp wondered how much longer their captivity would last. They longed for news of the war or any updates from home. Something to give them a flash of light, an assurance their lives in the prison camp weren't all they had left in this world.

Dorothy craned her neck, trying to look over the crowd. The commander at Los Baños allowed inmates to receive care packages from family members abroad. After a thorough search, the packages were ready for distribution. The inmates stood hopefully, eager to hear their names called. The Americans, particularly, were anxious for a piece of mail. A few weeks prior, a set of letters had arrived in the camp. As the stack of envelopes dwindled, disappointed Americans realized the letters were only for the British prisoners.

The previous autumn, the commander had grudgingly agreed to a Red Cross offer to deliver prisoners' letters to the United States. Months later, the inmates were still waiting for a response, unaware that the Red Cross mailing instructions were confusing and could result in delays of up to a year. At the time, Dorothy had written a letter to her parents, using large block letters the censors could easily read. The letter made it sound as though she was at boarding school. She began by telling her parents she missed them but assured them she was being "treated quite well." She described setting up the hospital under "amusing conditions" and teaching volunteers the fundamentals of nursing. "I enjoy it very much and find even in an internment camp many benefits can be derived." She revealed her conversion to Catholicism and how it had been a help and filled her "wanton life." Her words were carefully chosen to ensure that the letter would arrive uncensored. At home, inmates' families received advice on how to interpret such letters and respond accordingly. The inmates were not permitted to criticize their captors, so complaints were coded. The word *wanton* was likely interpreted by the censors as "meaningless" or "aimless." But it also meant cruel and malicious.

Inmates' families learned they also had to write with double meaning. Letters could not include any military references or news about the war. One navy physician imprisoned at a labor camp in Japan received a letter from his wife that referenced his son as a "happy youngster." The censors assumed the reference was to their young child. But the husband knew how to interpret the phrase. In his absence, his son had been accepted to the US Naval Academy and advanced to his second, or "youngster" year. Other families with sons who joined the military simply described them as absent, traveling, or gone for a while.

Dorothy heard her name called and eagerly accepted the package. She also had a letter, and she read the envelope as she walked from the crowd. The date was from early 1943, nearly a year ago. She opened the letter first. The Red Cross had instructed her mother to write vaguely and not reveal any military affiliations, so Arissa Still described the family as all doing well. They were thinking of painting the house a new color, and her sister and nephew were fine. They did not see her brother-in-law very much anymore. It took Dorothy several readings to realize that her brother-in-law was now a soldier fighting in the war.

Dorothy next tore into the package. Before sending it, her mother had received several letters from repatriated Americans who described life in the camps, so she knew not to trust the sunny newspaper stories about inmates taking culture classes and enjoying fresh meat. Everything she included in the package filled a practical need—white cotton pajamas, two toothbrushes, toothpaste, a printed blouse, underwear, and socks. Dorothy was overwhelmed with gratitude. She smoothed the clean fabrics between her fingers. It had been years since she felt fresh cotton socks. Before the war, the nurses typically wore white tights that stretched up to their knees. After internment, the best they could do was to knit socks for themselves using twine that had been unraveled into thin threads and then stitched into scratchy footwear.

Dorothy found her friend Thomas to share her good news. He also had received a package from home. She watched as he happily opened the box. His face lit up as he unwrapped his favorite pipe and a stash of tobacco, packed by his wife. His *wife*, Dorothy remembered. She thought of a warning she'd received from the camp priest. The priest encouraged her to befriend a Catholic bachelor in the camp, not a married man. Dorothy had assured the priest Thomas was just a good friend, but the priest sensed the young nurse was likely to be heartbroken when the arrangement inevitably ended.

"I wouldn't like to see you get hurt," the priest cautioned gently.

The priest's warning replayed in Dorothy's mind as she watched Thomas scrape the pipe bowl with a pocketknife. She envisioned him at home in California, sitting in the backyard and puffing on his pipe. She understood she would never be part of that scene. Shaken by the realization, Dorothy actively avoided Thomas the next few days. She did not meet him on the baseball diamond for their nightly star gaze, and she busied herself with a lengthy list of chores intended to distract her from the pain of ending the relationship. Thomas sensed the conflict, and confronted Dorothy about her distance. She agreed to speak with him, and the pair walked down a long path the prisoners defiantly called "Roosevelt Road."

Dorothy struggled to explain herself to Thomas. After a few incomplete sentences that ended in a pause and restarted with a new thought, she steadied herself and told Thomas the priest did not approve of their friendship. Thomas was a married man, Dorothy reminded him. Thomas resisted the logic. Did the priest oppose all friendships with the opposite sex if a person was married? Or did he just oppose Dorothy's friendship with Thomas?

The priest was specifically against Dorothy and Thomas as friends, she clarified. "He doesn't want to see me get hurt," she added.

Thomas looped his arm through Dorothy's and drew her close. He held her hand and looked directly into her eyes. Fate had thrown the two of them into the same prison camp. Their lives were forcefully paused by the war, and he knew their friendship was a type of "interlude." But Dorothy gave his life purpose and he needed her. Dorothy remained silent as Thomas described how she made him feel. She was essentially his anchor in the camp. She stopped him from drifting away.

Dorothy was quiet. Thomas looked at her seriously. "Has it ever occurred to you that we might not come out of this alive?"

Dorothy began to cry. Thomas pulled her into a hug. They held each other as Dorothy sobbed into his shirt and Thomas tried to soothe her. He wiped her tears and apologized for upsetting her. Dorothy pressed her cheek against his chest and listened to his heartbeat. She wasn't afraid to die. It had indeed occurred to her that she might not come out alive. She was more afraid of coming out alive and then losing the man she loved.

Peg Nash had more projects to coyly suggest to her carpenter friend. Another set of inmates were scheduled for transfer from Santo Tomas, and the infirmary needed to expand. The nurses were forfeiting their dormitory and squeezing into the infirmary basement. They were not keen on returning to such tight quarters, but their dormitory was ideal to serve as a ward. Peg was the resident interior designer among the nurses, and even Chief Nurse Cobb deferred to her ideas on how to improve the space. Peg hopefully mentioned to her carpenter friend that it would be nice to build the nurses a covered patio with a wooden floor. The carpenter agreed, and even added a wooden dining table.

The nurses were impressed with his craftsmanship. Mary Chapman ran her hand over the table's smooth surface. It reminded her of a picnic table. Perhaps, she suggested hopefully, when the war was over, the women could get together for a reunion and have a picnic. Mary's mind likely returned to her home in Chicago and the thought of warm summer evenings in the city parks. The other nurses looked at her in disbelief. When they got home, they were never eating *outside* again.

In the coming weeks, the table served other purposes. Dietitian Bertha Evans continued to have difficulty sleeping. She often woke up in the middle of the night, riddled with anxieties. She crept from the nurses' rooms to the patio and sat at the table. She listened to the quiet of the camp and looked up at the stars, thinking of her fiancé and her home in Oregon, and wondering if she'd ever see either again.

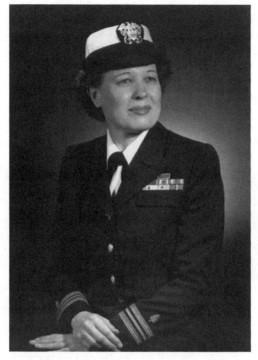

Navy nurse Bertha Evans. *Courtesy of Bureau of Medicine and Surgery*

Without news of the war, she did not know that help was indeed coming. Allied forces were advancing toward the Philippines, and the South Pacific was beginning to change. The Japanese Imperial Army was losing its grip on the islands south of the Philippines, near Australia. The Allied forces had reclaimed the Solomon Islands in early 1944 and turned their ambitions toward New Guinea. General MacArthur had landed his forces on New Guinea, and then in a move reminiscent of how the Japanese cut off Allied supplies in 1942, MacArthur strangled the supply chain so that twenty-five thousand Japanese troops had to either starve or surrender.

In March 1944, the Japanese military began seeing intensive losses. Air raids in New Guinea decimated their troops. It was all part of a new operation that isolated Japan by neutralizing or seizing area islands, while paying close attention to New Guinea. The Allies would then move up to the southern Philippine islands of Mindanao and Leyte.

Now, regaining the southern islands began to look possible. It would take a few months and bring intense fighting. But MacArthur planned to take back Manila and send a strong message to the Japanese emperor that he had returned.

Californian Margaret Sherk was anxious as she passed through the gate into Los Baños. She had volunteered to transfer from Santo Tomas with her six-year-old son, David, and infant daughter, Gerry Ann. The baby's father, Chicagoan Gerald Sams, had been transferred to the new camp almost eleven months earlier. She wrote to him when she learned she was pregnant, and a smuggled response promised he loved her. But almost a year had passed, and she did not know what she still meant to Gerald. The couple would soon be reunited—assuming they were still a couple.

Margaret was in a love triangle. Her husband, Bob, was a prisoner of war at the notorious Cabanatuan prison camp. He had learned of his wife's affair through an apologetic note in which Margaret confessed that the relationship had produced a child. A courier snuck him the message, and Margaret eventually received a response. Her husband forgave her and sidestepped her offer to quietly divorce after liberation. He wanted the war to be over, and if he survived Cabanatuan, he wanted to reunite with his wife and son.

Margaret was grateful for Bob's forgiveness, and she appreciated his kindness. But she still wanted a divorce. She burned for Gerald and had eagerly awaited the opportunity to relocate to Los Baños. Her opportunity came in April, when the commander announced the transfer of more than five hundred prisoners. She entered the camp hesitantly, wondering if Gerald still wanted her or if she was facing her own rejection.

Inmates circled the unloading trucks, eager to reunite with friends and family. It took a moment for Margaret to find Gerald in the sea of hopeful faces. He pushed his way to the truck and reached for her. Margaret was pleased—they were indeed still a couple. Rather, they were a *family*. The guards, however, would not allow the foursome to occupy the same cubicle. Family barracks were reserved for married couples only. In her mind, Margaret romantically thought of them as a forbidden family.

Margaret was relieved to be with Gerald, but she was horrified by the new camp and its lack of sanitation. The toilets were particularly disgusting, and although the Los Baños inmates were pleased with themselves for developing a way to flush the trough, Margaret was repulsed by the flies and the filth. And there was no toilet paper. The inmates had taken to using book pages to wipe themselves. Shakespeare, Margaret learned, was most prized, because the pages were thin and softer on the skin. The facilities made her think the Los Baños inmates were living like animals. Then she considered that wild animals probably lived in better conditions. They weren't trapped with the stench of their own filth.

Margaret was a quiet inmate who didn't bother others. In fact, she was more concerned with how other inmates perceived her. She kept her cubicle as clean as possible. She didn't steal or cut in line. The same could not be said for the other transfers. Margaret was one of the few new arrivals who had volunteered for reassignment to Los Baños. The nurses thought the Santo Tomas inmates had heard about the relentless mud and primitive facilities and wanted to stay put. They suspected that the executive committee had drafted their most undesirable inmates for transfer. Known thieves, gamblers, and prostitutes were put on the list. The executive committee also used the transfer as an opportunity to rid their camp of mental health patients.

The infirmary was soon at capacity, and the twelve nurses were managing almost two hundred patients a day. The administrative committee, meanwhile, was handling an influx of complaints about the new arrivals with criminal tendencies. Thieves waded into the inmates' gardens and helped themselves to eggplants and onions. Anyone caught with stolen vegetables was referred to the Court of Order, which soon learned that the camp degenerates weren't the only ones compelled to raid vegetable patches. The surgeon, Dana Nance, accused some nuns of stealing from his garden. The case went before the court with Thomas serving as the judge. Thomas dismissed the case after one of the surgeon's witnesses admitted he couldn't tell the nuns apart. In their habits, they all looked the same. Dorothy avoided the conflict. She was Catholic and felt a loyalty to the nuns. She resented Dana for accusing them, but she also appreciated him for always being on call, ready to serve his patients whenever needed.

There was a growing strain among the medical personnel, and she hadn't the energy to involve herself. The nurses were packed too tightly in the basement, and they irritated each other with their differences. Dorothy had a friend on the housing committee and she put in a request to transfer to the barracks. Eldene Paige was eager to join her as her roommate.

The request was quickly granted. Dorothy and Eldene were overjoyed to learn they were assigned a cubicle in one of the barracks that actually had four walls and a door. They were amazed to have the space just for the two of them. Of course, the wooden paneling was thin and noise drifted easily. But not having to *see* the other inmates was a respite. They felt for the first time in more than two years as though they had a shard of privacy, and that gave them a large dose of dignity. But they weren't truly alone in their cubicle. Insects scurried throughout the room and lizards followed the prey. There were times Dorothy locked eyes with a lizard lounging on her bed rail or trunk. She didn't appreciate having the creatures in her room, but she was also conditioned to no longer care.

13

I Have Returned

IN JULY 1944, the Japanese Imperial Army decided the inmates at
Los Baños had it too easy. Never mind that they lived among
vermin without modern plumbing, that they sheltered in hastily
constructed barracks and depended on vegetable gardens to supplement meager meals, or that they were emaciated and ravaged with
skin lesions. Despite all this, they were living too well for the army's
liking. The commander was accused of leniency and relieved of his
post. A new commander, Major Yasuaka Iwanaka, was assigned to
the position.

The inmates questioned whether Iwanaka was senile. The major
did not speak much English, and it was through his mannerisms
the inmates determined his memory was failing. He opted out of
military dress and instead shuffled around the camp in a kimono
and sandals. He seemed very relaxed by his surroundings and used
his time at Los Baños to focus on his artistic pursuits. The inmates
often saw him standing thoughtfully behind an easel, soaking in the
mountain view he wanted to capture in watercolor. Or they saw him
sitting quietly with a pen and paper, thinking about the next line in

his haiku. Iwanaka also appreciated the beauty of a potted plant and tended to geraniums as well as a small garden near his office.

With the commander disinterested in—or incapable of—running the camp, opportunity presented itself for a power-hungry officer to step into the void. Warrant Officer Sadaaki Konishi transferred to Los Baños in August and quickly sensed he could control the camp *his* way. He preferred meager food rations, limited space, and no outside assistance. Konishi wanted to put his boot on the entire camp and press down slowly.

Dorothy and the other inmates knew Konishi from Santo Tomas, where he had served as the supply officer. Or, more accurately, lack-of-supply officer. He cruelly rejected food deliveries and donations for thinly veiled reasons. One meat delivery, he claimed, had to be denied because the truck did not show up on time. There was no reasoning with the man, and the inmates remembered him as an angry guard who demanded complete submission. He slapped inmates for unpredictable reasons, including bowing improperly to guards. Only deep bows initiated from the hips, not the waist, were acceptable.

In his two years at Santo Tomas, Konishi clashed with the civilian commanders, who had a more benign approach to internment. After the civilian commanders were booted from Santo Tomas in early 1944, Konishi found more success with the army officers. The camp became more filthy, desperate, violent—just as he wanted. There were inmates who intentionally moved to Los Baños to escape Konishi, and they were devastated to hear of his arrival.

Dorothy was also distressed. She thought he was a sadistic man who tormented the inmates for his own amusement. On one occasion, he ordered inmates to move five hundred sacks of rice from the guards' storage facility to the inmates' storage facility, and then promptly ordered them to move everything back. He was so pleased with watching the defeated inmates return rice they could not eat that he revisited the trick at a later date. Once again, the inmates moved hundreds of bags to their storage facility only to be told to lug it back. The inmates refused, and Konishi ordered the guards to repossess the rice.

Konishi replaced the rice bag hoax with another ploy that didn't require his guards to heave heavy bags. On multiple occasions, he alerted the kitchen staff to expect a delivery of a thousand pounds of sweet potatoes or beans. The crew excitedly prepared only to receive a paltry two-hundred-pound delivery, most of which was rotten.

The man was mean, and the campers wondered why. Rumors about his past life were spun throughout the camp. Some heard he was injured in the Manchurian campaign. Others heard he was a rural farmer without an education. His age was heavily debated. Konishi was actually twenty-seven, but many inmates assumed he was at least a decade older. His skin was weathered from his alcoholism as well as his incessant smoking.

Konishi's smoking stained his teeth and fingers a tobacco-brown color the inmates found repulsive. They were also disgusted by his lack of hygiene. The guards had access to showers and laundry, yet Konishi wore the same shirt for days. Sweat stains circled under his armpits and then dried, leaving behind a dark ring. The next day, a new circle formed and bled down the side of the shirt, leaving another ring. The inmates surmised the number of rings were indicative as to how many days in a row he'd worn the same shirt.

Despite his foul clothing and stained teeth, Konishi was convinced of his own superiority. He was indoctrinated in the army's belief of Japanese racial superiority, and he had little tolerance for other Asian cultures. Proponents of Japanese supremacy believed that Japan should dominate Asia. They cast other Asian cultures, particularly the Chinese and Koreans, as "backward" societies worthy of violence. Similarly, Europeans and white North Americans were "pigs" who needed to recognize their own inferiority.

Japan's early dominance in the war reaffirmed Konishi's conviction regarding Japanese preeminence. But Allied resistance steadily mounted, and in the fall of 1944 Japan suffered heavy naval losses. Konishi responded by cutting the camp's food rations by 20 percent. He also banned inmates from possessing money, trading with locals, or receiving deliveries. They were now completely dependent on the two meals served by the camp kitchen.

One inmate thought confiscating money was how the Japanese finally broke their captives' morale. Ethel Chapman was imprisoned with her husband at Santo Tomas and observed the many collective humiliations pressed on the inmates. Each time, Ethel saw a resilience in the human spirit. The commander, for example, once insisted that every inmate submit to a photograph for record keeping. He assumed the photograph would bring the inmates great disgrace. But these were people who had been defecating in front of each other for years. The guards wouldn't be able to shame them with a mug shot. Another time, the commander compelled inmates to provide personal histories including birthplace and most recent address. The inquiry was intended to feel violating, and the inmates developed a subtle resistance. The Americans responded amiably to the questions, and then tried to outdo each other by giving ridiculous street names and fictitious hometowns. But the loss of money, Ethel thought, finally crushed their spirits. They were truly dependent on a commander prepared to show no mercy.

———————

Bertha Evans stood outside the infirmary, looking up toward the bright blue sky. A plane soared in the distance. Bertha focused on the low-flying plane jetting toward the camp. She thought she saw a white star—the distinctive American marking—on the tail. She watched intently as the plane flew past and felt a swelling in her chest. The US

Army was back! Bertha had to stop herself from waving. The guards did not tolerate an inmate trying to communicate with their enemy. But she felt satisfied in knowing the Americans knew they were there. She felt as though the pilot had communicated by tipping the wing, as if he was saying, *Hold on. We are coming for you.*

The Americans actually did not yet know that Los Baños existed. Only in December would a young major from California hear about the camp in passing. The major was in Manila on an intelligence mission, interviewing a local from a southern island who had gone up to the capital to secure medication for his wife. The man mentioned that on his way home, he would be passing the big POW camp—the one with the American civilians. The major was stunned to learn that more than two thousand civilians lived in the camp and they were in desperate conditions.

The Los Baños inmates sensed Allied forces were nearby, which meant the war was beginning to change. In the middle of September, they felt the ground vibrate from bombs. But more so, they felt the aftershocks of American advancement through Konishi. In September and October, he again cut food rations so inmates received an average of eight hundred calories per day. He halted garden operations and ordered that the vegetables be left to rot in the fields, even though some were ripe for picking. Then he reduced inmates' space and insisted the guards cut off parts of the campus with barbed wire. His superior continued with his watercolors.

Dorothy keenly felt all the deprivations. She twice asked nurse Goldia to take in inches from her uniform. And she stopped having periods due to the weight loss. She was confused for several weeks, uncertain as to why she had missed her cycle. She confided in Bertha, who had undergone a hysterectomy due to uterine tumors. Dorothy wondered if she had developed the same condition. Bertha was almost impatient with her response: nearly all the women were so emaciated they no longer had a menstrual cycle. Dorothy had been one of the final holdouts.

No longer having a period struck Dorothy as a blessing. In a camp with no running water or sanitation, it was difficult to manage monthly bleeding. The camp didn't have toilet paper, let alone sanitary napkins. The women had to rinse and reuse fabric swatches. The filthy process put them at risk for yeast and urinary tract infections, both of which the infirmary could do little to alleviate.

Starvation relieved women of their periods, but it also brought on a distressing condition. Incontinence was a camp-wide problem toward the end of 1944. Losing control of the bladder was a side effect that many inmates did not expect until they experienced a sudden burst of urine. Typically, the urge to urinate happened at the same time as the release. It often occurred at night, forcing the inmate to remain in soaked sheets until after the morning headcount. And as energy dwindled, the prospect of washing bedding seemed more than a weakened person could handle.

Many of the debilitated inmates tended only to their own personal needs. But the nurses continued to work despite their severe malnourishment. With more than two hundred patients coming to the infirmary each day, the women had to put in twelve-hour shifts. They moved slowly and deliberately, amazed at how profoundly their bodies had changed. Actions that had once been easy were now a challenge the nurses had to think through. The nurses all developed a chronic shaking in their hands that made it difficult to give injections. Patients watched uncomfortably as a nurse with trembling hands tried to find a strong vein and then unsteadily pressed a needle into their skin.

Tumbling and tripping became a regular occurrence in the infirmary. Weakened orderlies tried to push beds but then lost strength in their legs and collapsed to the floor. Nurses bending over a patient found they did not have the back muscles to right themselves. And staff who squatted next to a patient bed flopped to the ground when their quads were too debilitated to push them upright.

Some of the patients felt sympathy toward the medical staff for continuing to work even though they had their own ailments. But others seemed to think the nurses were there to serve them, and Dorothy often felt frustrated with their lack of gratitude. One mother, whose young son had fallen from a tree he shouldn't have been climbing, was irritated when Dana Nance was not present to examine the injury. The medical staff thought his swollen leg was sprained, but the mother was convinced her boy had a broken bone. Before leaving that evening, she instructed the nurse at the front desk to have the doctor look at her son as soon as he returned to the infirmary. She was confident he would agree with her diagnosis.

It was the type of civilian expectation that annoyed the nurses. The infirmary lacked an X-ray machine, so there was no way of knowing whether the bone was broken or the injury was a sprain. Regardless of the diagnosis, the treatment was the same. They didn't have plaster of paris, so they couldn't cast the limb. They had to keep the boy in the hospital for three days until they could fashion a leg brace from rubber. The brace was removed after six weeks, and the mother again irritated the medical staff with her expectations. She had anticipated a full recovery. Instead, her son limped painfully for two months. She was critical of the outcome; it seemed as though she felt the medical staff had failed to properly serve her family.

But the infirmary had more pressing cases to address. Within a few months of Konishi's arrival, inmates began to die of starvation and neglect. American Irving Posner was one of the first to die, shortly after his sixty-ninth birthday. A native of New York, he had lived in the Philippines for decades. After the Japanese occupation, he was accused of being a spy and subjected to the Kempeitai, the Japanese version of the Gestapo. Irving was held for six months at Fort Santiago, a dungeon-like citadel where the Kempeitai tortured suspected spies.

Irving told others that he didn't experience the worst of Fort Santiago. But his stories made listeners rethink the depths of human cruelty. He spoke of being interrogated while hot coils of metal were pressed against his bare feet. He also told of the Kempeitai's dreaded water torture. Gallons of water were poured down his throat as guards jumped on his stomach and forced the water back up. Irving had suffered severe damage to his kidneys, bladder, and intestines.

The Kempeitai accused Irving of being a member of the Freemasons; they believed the secret society had the potential to undermine the occupation with their covert ways. The torture continued until Irving's captors realized he wasn't a Freemason, he was Jewish. An interrogator looked into Irving's watery gray eyes and decided the two of them were kindred spirits. The Jews were reviled in Europe, and the interrogator, feeling that the Japanese had also been subject to white imperialism, was sympathetic to their plight. Irving was stunned— the Japanese killed *millions* of civilians, mostly Asians they viewed as inferior. They occupied China and Korea. And they were aligned with Germany, the country driving the genocide against Jews. But Irving was not about to correct the man willing to release him from extreme torture. Irving nodded in agreement and was transferred to the civilian camp at Los Baños the next day.

Malnutrition shredded Irving's feeble body. Dana sat for hours with Irving during his final weeks, listening to him talk about his life in the Philippines and the suffering he had experienced at Fort Santiago. Listening was a graciousness that history would fail to show the other Fort Santiago survivors. The stories were so brutal that the inhumanity was impossible for the average person to comprehend. But Dana had seen the brutality of war, and in Irving's final days, he gave his fellow prisoner the gift of being heard.

Several older patients followed Irving to the camp cemetery. Two Americans in their early sixties passed away, and then a Catholic nun. The patients in their sixties had outlived the life expectancy for someone born before 1880, but that was cold comfort to the nurses. They knew the victims had died of starvation, disease, and complications from torture. Their deaths—no matter their advanced age—were unnecessary. The deceased were lowered into coffins and buried in the thick mud while clergy prayed and mourners cried angrily.

Emotions peaked after the death of a kind young inmate. Twenty-year-old Burton Fonger died from malaria. The parasite had advanced quickly into his brain, and for days, the infirmary staff devoted round-the-clock care to their effort to save him. His death devastated many in the camp. The young people in particular reeled from the sudden void in their lives. Burt had been active with a group of teenagers who called themselves the "Class of '47." He helped build the camp orchestra by copying music by hand and then organizing young musicians to meet on the camp playground. Any instruments they had with them in the camp were in disrepair, and the teenagers seemed too defeated to play with cracked reeds and broken strings. But Burt banged on his snare drum and the other musicians eventually joined in, touched by his enthusiasm. And then he was gone.

Streams of inmates staggered to the chapel for the funeral service. A woman from Ohio named Grace Nash played the violin, as requested by Burton's mother. But as Grace lifted her bow to play "Ave Maria," she was crippled with a sense of defeat. Burton had been part of all the small things the inmates did to feel like they weren't just surviving, they were living. Now that he was gone, Grace thought the rest of them were doomed. She no longer saw a point to living or even trying. Konishi was slowly starving them all to death.

Grace looked out at the hillside where the youngest members of the camp had come to say good-bye to a young man who was like their big brother. Were they all to die? Grace felt tears spill down her cheeks. Her hand holding her bow quivered. What was the use of trying anymore?

But then she thought of the young man who had once roused teenagers to play broken instruments. She realized they had to move forward. They had to take a chance on living. Konishi was trying to kill them, but the inmates had to resolve to live. Grace lifted her bow and began to play.

In late October, the nurses still didn't know much about life outside Los Baños. They had seen several warplanes and they sensed the power dynamic tilting toward the Allied forces. But they did not know that US forces had landed on Leyte, a Philippine island several hundred miles to the southeast of Manila. For the United States, it was time for retribution. MacArthur menacingly announced, "I have returned," and intended to crush the enemy. The Japanese Imperial Army sensed he had the ability to do so, and began plotting its own evacuation. The Allies controlled the skies, had decimated the Japanese naval fleet, and were now coming by land.

But the Japanese army was not willing to leave their able-bodied prisoners behind. Within weeks of being liberated, former prisoners could be fed, medicated, and turned into fighting machines on a mission for revenge. Imperial Army officials strategized how to transport military prisoners to Japan to work in factories, farms, mines, and mills. They began moving thousands of men from the Cabanatuan prison camp down to Manila and then onto the "hell ships" destined for Japan. The Japanese army did not care if their human cargo survived; all that mattered was they were ferried from the islands and kept far from rescuers. Dorothy didn't know that her corpsmen from Cavite were on those "hell ships," and that the men she'd once called her brothers were in the final miserable days of their lives.

Dorothy had to wonder if she herself was in the final days of her life. Konishi seemed to be on a rampage, and every few days brought a new limitation designed to slowly kill the inmates. Contact between guards and inmates, for example, was now forbidden, in order to prevent sympathetic guards from helping the prisoners. The camp commander remained oblivious. He padded around the grounds in his slippers and tried to engage Japanese speakers in pleasant conversations about music or art. He used his limited English skills to make a bizarre, false promise to inmates. "You will have a nice Christmas," he assured.

Optimistic inmates assumed the commander meant he was overriding Konishi and allowing in Red Cross comfort kits. Hungry inmates began debating the contents of the kits. Would there be a corned beef tin this year? What about the margarine packet? Would the comfort kit also include the sanitation kit with soap or toilet paper, or might that be a separate delivery?

Dorothy and the other nurses prayed for the comfort kits. The inmates needed nutrition and the infirmary needed medicine. Inmates were coming in droves to the infirmary with wet beriberi, a vitamin B deficiency that caused swollen joints and puffed limbs. Others had urinary tract infections after years of standing for hours in toilet lines. The nurses had little to offer the patients. Even the home remedies were in short supply.

In the three months since his arrival, Konishi had brought the entire camp population to the brink of death. Comfort kits, if allowed, would help the inmates survive a few more weeks. But what the camp truly needed was liberation. The nurses sensed the Allies were close. They just didn't know how long they could last.

14

Do the Best You Can

VIOLENCE AND DEATH permeated the camp in the last two months of 1944. At the infirmary, Dorothy and the other nurses tended to a woman in the throes of the advanced stages of wet beriberi, well beyond responding to the infirmary's vitamin B tablets. The swelling had advanced from her hands and feet into her limbs. Her stomach plumped and then her torso. Dorothy was struck with how quickly the emaciated woman bloated into the shape of a morbidly obese person. The woman met a violent end. Her neck and tongue swelled, and she gasped for air as fluid filled her lungs. The nurses watched helplessly as the woman writhed in suffocation. Her misery ended when her heart failed.

The nurses also saw patients suffering the remnants of earlier assaults. One American man had been beaten so brutally by guards at Fort Santiago that his collarbone punctured the top of his lung. A British internee had a deep leg wound that ran from his ankle to his knee. The man's crime, Dorothy learned, was trying to send food to the prisoners in the military camps. A sentry slashed his leg as punishment. Some of the injuries were years old, but the pain continued to taunt the prisoners daily.

Other wounds were recently acquired. A Philadelphian at Los Baños was slapped so hard across the face that he temporarily lost his hearing. The inmate had been tasked with leaving the supply list on the commander's desk on behalf of the camp. He knew to bow before entering, but he saw the office was empty and assumed he was not obligated to bow to an unoccupied desk. He was confronted outside by an angry lieutenant. The officer ferociously slapped the man, bloodying his nose and mouth, and damaging his ear.

Anyone near the commander's office saw the inmate beaten by the lieutenant. On other occasions, the guards deliberately summoned an audience for a punishment in order to traumatize the other inmates. One woman was struck with a sword after a guard claimed she did not properly bow. A crowd of horrified inmates was forced to watch as the woman was ordered to bow fifty times.

The guards were not the only ones in the camp who inflicted violence. All the civilian POW camps contained nasty inmates who intimidated meek prisoners with the threat of violence. The aggressors accused their victims of small slights and then stared antagonistically in the dormitories, letting the target know that today might indeed be the day they unleashed their fury. Others simply reacted violently when something did not go their way. One American woman at Los Baños attacked the head of the housing committee after he decided she must share her cubicle. The woman launched herself onto the man's back and scratched his face, creating long bloody lines across the skin. The situation was resolved only after the threat of involving Konishi prompted her to accept the new roommate on a temporary basis. And at Santo Tomas, one woman was hospitalized after an inmate in her dormitory savagely beat her without warning. The aggressor had severe mental issues, and the other inmates agreed the attack was unprovoked. They also sensed there was nothing they could do to punish the perpetrator without involving the commanders.

Children in the camp also dealt with aggression. Small children were targets of angry older kids who were stressed by prison life or just flat-out mean. Grace Nash encouraged her two older sons to stay together so they might avoid the camp bully who had once choked her four-year-old boy. The tormentor had squeezed the boy's neck until a passing adult stopped the strangulation. For days, the boy couldn't swallow or talk without pain.

Even the few domesticated animals in the camp were subject to violence. Cats were lured into traps and used for food. Most pet dogs had died from malnutrition, with the exception of Poochie, a Labrador mix whose mere existence made Dana Nance feel murderous. Poochie belonged to an American family who had long resided in Los Baños before the war. The father was once a professor at the university and was now relegated to living in a barrack just yards away from his former classroom. The professor was interned along with his wife, two sons in their early twenties, a daughter and her husband, and a brother-in-law. The daughter and her husband fed Poochie from their own rations; they took from no one to keep the dog alive. Yet watching the dog eat a small plate of rice enraged Dana. He wanted the sixty-pound dog dead and in a cooking pot.

Before Thanksgiving, Dana grabbed a surgical knife and went hunting for the dog. Someone saw the doctor dragging the dog behind the infirmary, knife in hand, and went running for the professor's sons. The young men were swollen thick with wet beriberi but hustled toward the infirmary to stop the slaying. They were too late. Dana had already slit the dog's neck and was slicing open the stomach.

The young men lunged at Dana. They were significantly taller than the doctor but in far worse condition. They succeeded in breaking his glasses and bloodying his nose, but then Dana was able to push them off. He retreated from the scene as the guards approached, leaving the dog carcass with its weeping owners. The young men vowed that Dana would not eat their dog. They smeared insecticide on Poochie and buried her near the barbed wire.

Dorothy and the other nurses did not respect Dana's attack on the dog. She had to admit he was not as well fed as he once had been, but he was in better condition than the rest of the camp. Dana had negotiated a larger share of rations for himself, arguing that as a medical care provider he needed more food than others. He was adept at securing his own food sources, and hunting Poochie seemed like another attempt at a caloric windfall for himself, not a heroic attempt to feed others. At the infirmary, the nurses mocked Dana and joked that despite the poison, he probably still had plans to craft a meal from the dead dog. They half expected him to dig up the bones and boil them in a broth.

Dana might have been ashamed by his sudden surge of savagery. Or he might have been relieved to no longer see the dog in the camp. It pained him to see the dog live while people were dying in the infirmary from starvation. One man gave most of his rations to his family and then died of malnutrition. Another inmate died after trying to eat his belt. Desperate inmates stared at the coconuts and bananas growing on the other side of the barbed wire. They cringed and stuffed leaves and insects into their mouths instead.

Dana expected the situation to intensify in the coming weeks. The small scoops of mush the inmates received twice daily had almost no nutritional value. Half the camp had symptoms of clinical malnutrition, and more than a hundred people had severe vitamin deficiency.

Four hundred people reported to the infirmary with wet or dry beri-beri. While the wet version swelled the body and then attacked the cardiovascular system, the dry version compromised the nervous system while making the patient resemble a walking skeleton. Both conditions could be solved with vitamins, but the infirmary had a scant stash. The camp was out of most supplies, even the makeshift versions. Homemade soap was no longer possible to concoct without lard or coconut oil. And the tree that produced sap had been chopped down for firewood, so the pharmacists could no longer make bandage adhesive.

Chief Nurse Cobb encouraged her nurses. "Do the best you can," she repeated. She reminded them of the American planes spotted in the skies. She urged them to believe liberation was coming soon.

Dorothy made the conscious decision to appear bright for the patients. She didn't feel cheerful but she smiled at the men and women in her ward. She realized all those patients had in that moment was a nurse who cared. They didn't have medicine or supplies. They didn't have food or privacy. They had only a smiling nurse who made them feel they had a reason to continue living. She maintained a pleasant expression, even when she learned Konishi had blocked the comfort kits. He also refused a food donation from the Vatican. It was not, as the commander once promised, going to be a good Christmas.

Margaret Sherk didn't think she was going to make it until Christmas. She was admitted into the infirmary with a searing pain in her side. Dana diagnosed appendicitis, but Margaret said her appendix had been removed years earlier. Nevertheless, she submitted to an operation. With a shaky scalpel, Dana cut into her lower stomach and found that indeed her appendix had been removed. He suspected the pain was the result of tuberculosis of the lower bowel, a condition that typically afflicted impoverished people with compromised immune systems.

All Dana could do was sew up the incision. Margaret's recovery was slow, and it was hindered by her need to nurse her baby every four hours. Margaret was forty pounds underweight, and she produced little milk for her daughter. She felt depressed watching her daughter frantically try to feed, and she dreaded seeing the child's father appear at the infirmary door with their hungry baby. Margaret lost her will to live. She wanted to close her eyes and never wake up. She wished for death, but it did not come for her. It was, however, coming for others.

———————

Prisoner Rufus W. Smith didn't want to get into the trench. The twenty-six-year-old marine preferred to stay above ground during air raids and watch American planes soar over the prison camp. Rufus was being held captive on Palawan, an island southwest of Manila. He had surrendered at Corregidor and then endured the Cabanatuan prison camp during the summer of 1942, where dysentery raged, killing dozens of men each day.

Wanting out of Cabanatuan, Rufus had heard the Japanese army was recruiting able-bodied men to transfer to a new camp. He asked for an American officer to put in a good word for him so that he might make the cut. It felt like good fortune when he was selected. There were only 150 men in the Palawan camp, and although their work promised to be intense, Rufus hoped it would be an improvement.

Instead, the new camp was a deeper level of hell. Cabanatuan prisoners had been forced onto work details, but there were thousands of men at the camp. At Palawan, there were only 150 prisoners, and a slave-master dynamic quickly developed. The prisoners were tasked with clearing trees for an airplane runway using only picks and shovels. The work was arduous, and the once able-bodied men deteriorated into a pack of tattered prisoners who were gaunt, rav-aged, and beaten regularly by guards who changed their expectations without warning.

Rufus and the other inmates had no recreation or leisure. They were devoid of energy after a long day of working in the hot sun. Rufus once got hold of a ball and considered organizing a game, until he realized he was too exhausted to play. In time, his entire existence was the airstrip. The prisoners eventually cleared an area the length of four city blocks and then, mixing cement by hand, surfaced the entire landing strip.

Toward the end of 1944, American forces began bombing the strip. The prisoners were sent into shallow trenches to wait out the air raid. They were then responsible for cleaning the debris from the airfield and patching the holes. The inmates were secretly delighted by the explosions, even though clearing rocks from the cratered airstrip was physically demanding. The bombings meant the Americans were on the attack, and the prisoners hoped liberation was near.

The guards at Palawan also sensed their position in the war was changing. Italy had surrendered, and it was expected Germany would soon follow suit. The Japanese directed their frustrations toward the inmates. The prisoners had always been subject to hard slaps, but now beatings became random and unpredictable. There were occasions when guards stormed into the barracks in the middle of the night and pummeled prisoners as they slept.

On the morning of December 14, Rufus and the other prisoners trudged to the airfield to repair bomb damage. Before lunch, they were ordered back to the camp, which struck the inmates as odd. Life for the previous two years had been painfully routine, and they always ate the midday meal at the airfield. But the guards claimed more Ameri-can planes were heading in their direction and they needed to take cover. Rufus resisted getting into the trench until a guard's bayonet tip persuaded him to climb into the shallow shelter.

The guards did not know they had shoved Rufus into a trench with an escape hatch. When the prisoners were excavating it, they'd hit coral and realized they could dig their way to the beach. The tunnel opened onto a cliff less than a hundred feet above the shore. The descent was traversable, and Rufus knew escape was possible. They had disguised the hatch with leaves and dirt. Rufus hoped to never have to use it.

Rufus huddled in the trench, waiting to hear the planes screech past. Deliverance, he hoped, was finally upon them. He heard screaming and gleefully thought Filipino resistance fighters were attacking the guards. Rufus's friend, Corporal Glenn "Mac" McDole, stood from the trench to see what was happening. It wasn't the Allies. Guards strode along the trenches with burning torches and buckets of gas. One of them hurled a torch into a trench, and a stream of gasoline followed.

The first trench ignited. Men screamed as they were engulfed in flames. Prisoners who tried to run from the inferno were hit by machine gun fire.

"My God, they are murdering everyone!" Mac yelled to Rufus.

Rufus commanded the men near the escape hatch to begin pushing out the cover. "All right, you guys. Get busy. Knock that side out!" Rufus ordered.

A torch flew into Rufus's trench, but for whatever reason the guard above failed to follow with the gasoline. At the other end, men scurried through the hatch and out onto the cliff.

"Mac, I got most of the fellows out of here," Rufus called to his friend.

"OK, I'm coming."

Mac and Rufus paused for a moment on the cliff above the beach. The guards were still ignorant of the tunnel, but now they could see the prisoners escaping through the barbed wire and speeding toward the shore. Rufus and Mac needed to quickly conceal themselves from the Japanese soldiers. They looked at the coral beach below. For three years, garbage had spilled from the camp and tumbled down the cliff. Some of the survivors were covering themselves with trash. Others hid behind large coral formations.

Rufus casually bid good-bye to his friend, as if he expected to see him in a short while. "Well, I'll see you."

Mac made his way down and covered himself in garbage. Rufus was a lanky man with long legs, and he nimbly scrambled down the cliff and burst across the beach to find a hiding spot. He momentarily huddled with four other men behind a jagged coral outcrop. But he sensed they would be too easy to find, and he broke from the group. He climbed higher onto the cliffs and lay down in a patch of tall grass.

For the next three hours, the guards hunted the survivors. Rufus heard screams from prisoners stabbed with bayonets or burned alive. One guard came within mere feet of Rufus, but the bright sun made it difficult for him to see that a prisoner lay in the grass. A few hours later, another patrol came through, stabbing the grass randomly to weed out hidden survivors. One of the guards stepped on Rufus but either didn't realize it or chose not to alert the others.

Rufus's heart pounded and he tried to control his breathing until the guards passed. After sunset, he eased himself down to the beach. Standing at the water's edge, he hesitated to enter the darkness, but he glanced back at the cliff and saw the silhouette of a guard. He had no choice. He silently slid under the water and began to swim. He surfaced, took a deep breath, and pushed himself under again.

Gaining distance from the garbage-strewn beach, he paddled in the dark, the salty water preventing him from opening his eyes underwater. But he could see he was not alone. The fish glowed with bioluminescence. Schools of them swam near, while solitary fish came close with curiosity and then darted away. Rufus's large moving shape soon attracted the attention of a sand shark. The long gray beast lunged at his shoulder and grabbed his flesh between its jagged teeth. Rufus pried the creature from his arm and the stunned shark swam away, realizing he was not easy prey. But the damage was more than the exhausted man could endure. He felt his way atop a nearby fishing trap and rested on the cage until he had the strength to resume swimming.

By the time he reached the other side of the bay, Rufus estimated he had swum at least five miles. For several hours, he lay flat on his back on the beach, trying to get the strength to stand. He finally steadied himself on the coral and climbed up the cliff to a small hut he sensed was occupied by Filipinos. The six men inside were indeed sympathetic to the tattered prisoner. They supplied him with food, water, and a change of clothes. They sent for a doctor to tend to his shark bite, and then gave him directions to the headquarters of the local resistance fighters.

Rufus was one of only eleven men to survive the Palawan massacre. Mac also survived by spending the night in the garbage pile and then swimming for an entire day. The men were now under the protection of the resistance fighters, but it took weeks for them to be evacuated from the island and taken into the custody of the US Army.

After the men's rescue, American military officials were horrified by the survivors' revelations, and the army considered rescuing inmates at other camps. It was decided Cabanatuan had to take precedence. The camp held survivors of the Bataan Death March, and the population had dwindled to five hundred men, a small enough group for the Japanese to quickly slaughter. Bilibid Prison and Santo Tomas were also considered feasible possibilities for liberation, given that the army intended to liberate Manila. Los Baños, however, was low priority, since capturing the area would not present the US Army with any type of strategic advantage. Dorothy and the other inmates at Los Baños would have to wait.

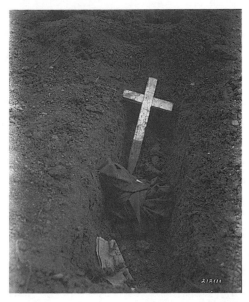

Allied forces buried the remains of prisoners who had been burned alive during the Palawan Massacre in December 1944. The massacre motivated the Allies to liberate other prison camps. *Courtesy of National Archives, https://catalog .archives.gov/id/531317*

On Christmas Day, Lieutenant Konishi strode through the camp with a satisfied smirk. He was making progress. The men in his camp looked terrible, more so than the woman. The men had lost body fat faster, and when they took their shirts off in the heat, Konishi saw the results of his work. Pectoral muscles now lay flat against torsos, and rib bones protruded from the clavicle down. The women's deterioration was hidden under blouses, skirts, and slacks, but their upper arms were typically as reed thin as their frail wrists. Their faces showed tight skin that wrinkled around the mouth when they tried to smile.

This was what Konishi wanted. The inmates were so lethargic and obsessed with food that they skipped their Christmas festivities from previous years. Some inmates did bring out tins of Spam they had saved for the occasion and invited neighbors or friends to join them. Grace Nash and her husband had two meat tins to share, which they spread among ten people, along with mush, greens, and papaya puree. The papayas had come from a compassionate guard who sold several pieces of Grace's jewelry on the outside and used the money to buy six pieces of fruit.

Dorothy spent the holiday with Thomas and her friend Eldene. Thomas had a squash to contribute to the meal. He had ventured near the gate, where a sympathetic local appeared and motioned him over. The man pushed the vegetable into his hands, and Thomas walked away nonchalantly. Dorothy contributed a tin of "party loaf" she had saved from the previous December's comfort kit. The three collected their mush from the chow line and then added the squash and the meat loaf, the latter of which had been fried in facial cold cream. It was a tasteless, bizarre meal, yet it was the best they would have for weeks to come.

Dorothy did have one nice surprise on Christmas Day. Thomas had traded his fountain pen with a guard in exchange for an entire roll of toilet paper. When he presented his gift to Dorothy, she could not believe the luxury. She likened it to receiving beautiful jewelry, except the roll of toilet paper was useful and therefore better. She strategized as to how she could make it last. She also had to consider whether she wanted to use it on the toilet, or if it might serve more practical purposes.

Dorothy attended midnight mass and listened to a choir of clergy sing favorite Christmas songs. She sat for the performance with a calm look on her face that concealed how she felt: the holiday brought a defeating gloom. This was her third Christmas in the camp, and the milestone felt miserable. Each time, she had expected the new year to bring liberation. It had yet to come, and now it seemed as though her life in California was beyond her reach. Five years had passed since she last saw her family or her homeland. She had to wonder whether if she'd see either again.

The milestone was also a reminder how her time in the camp had eaten away the expectations she set for her own life. She was meant to return to the United States on January 1, 1942. She'd seen herself getting married, perhaps to a naval officer, and starting a family. None of these things transpired. She had turned thirty at the end of November and felt she had nothing to show for it. Her prized possessions included a sliver of soap, the tin the party loaf came in, and a sketchbook the dentist had filled with funny caricatures of the hospital staff.

Reminders of the life that might have been appeared in years-old newspapers that were passed among the inmates. Newspaper reports about the war were never permitted in the camps, but sometimes internees got hold of a fashion page from an old American newspaper, showing the upcoming styles for seasons already long past. It had been three years since Dorothy had even thought about what colors and cuts would be fashionable in the new year. Seeing such news articles made her think of the life that was passing her by.

Memories of a past life also surfaced in the inmates' obsessive thoughts about food. Almost every conversation between inmates gravitated toward food, and sharing old recipes was now a dominant pastime. Inmates described to eager listeners how much flour they used to add to the batter or how long they would let the meat sear before flipping to the other side. Prisoners also collected recipes from books and magazines, especially prizing those with photos. Even Dorothy and the other nurses, who tried to stay busy and mentally occupied, found themselves having in-depth conversations about meal preferences.

As the inmates dreamed of old recipes and prepared their scant Christmas meals, the war in the Philippines raged on. On December 25, the Japanese abandoned organized resistance on the island of Leyte. They expected the Americans to advance to the main island of Luzon and capture Manila. In preparation, the Imperial Army had liquidated the Baguio prison camp north of the capital and sent the internees to Bilibid.

At Los Baños, Konishi refused to accept any possibility that the United States was advancing. He remained fervent in his belief that the Japanese would conquer the world. He supported the sudden replacement of Japanese guards with Formosans, Taiwanese aboriginals forced to serve Japan. By placing the Formosans between his soldiers and the inmates, Konishi hoped to convey the superiority of the Japanese race. But the inmates didn't interpret the message as the Imperial Army intended. To them, a guard was just a guard.

Part V

1945

15

'Tis You, 'Tis You Must Go and I Must Bide

DOROTHY HAD NEVER seen Chief Nurse Laura Cobb cry. Her commander had steeled herself through the worst of the war. At Cavite, Cobb rocketed between the wards wearing a purposeful look that concealed her dismay. Twice Dorothy had to swallow a sob, and once she went outside to weep. But Cobb seemed to think her own emotions were a luxury to which she was not entitled. She'd also denied her fear at Santa Scholastica, even when nurse Peg Nash was selected for execution. And when that crisis passed, she remained poised even though the Japanese Imperial Army planned to separate her nurses.

Cobb always stood a step ahead of her nurses. She herded her group together, pushing them back into position if anyone drifted. When Dorothy retched with hepatitis, it was Cobb who followed the young woman into the bathroom. And when Susie had her heart attack, it was Cobb whom the pained woman clutched as she stumbled to the hospital. Cobb approached her patients with the same resolve. She never cried when tearful inmates described the torture from which they had received their injuries. And she kept her emotions to herself when prisoners began dying from starvation and tropical diseases and the internment camp became a slow-processing death camp. If the navy nurses were the anchors of the camp, then Cobb was the mooring. The weight of her strength was heftier, and the woman had tremendous holding power.

Cobb now sat next to the bed of her close friend, Hugh Hosking Williams. She fought back the tears, but they slipped from her lower lids and splashed down her cheeks. Dorothy was stunned and a little frightened by her chief's emotions. In all the years they had been confined together, in all they had endured, Cobb had never shed a tear. Hugh's death broke her tenacity. Cobb needed that man and losing him collapsed her defenses.

Hugh was in his midsixties when he came to the infirmary with intense stomach pain. He suffered acute colitis from eating too many plants and roots. An intestinal blockage was killing him, and the medical staff worked to save their special patient. Dana Nance and the surgical team tried cutting into his abdomen to remove the obstruction. Cobb no doubt stood in the operating room, anxiously watching as nurse Susie held the gauze mask over her beloved's face. But Dana was at a loss. The damage had advanced beyond remedy.

Cobb remained at Hugh's bedside as he slipped from the world. Hugh was a New Zealander, born in the 1880s in Dunedin. He spent his life at sea, first with a steamship company and then with the navy during World War I. He had a wife and two children, but the couple separated after his wife refused to move up the coast to Auckland. Hugh later transferred to Hong Kong and started a new life on his own. His days as a sea captain ended while he was towing a British vessel to the safety of Singapore. The Japanese air force bombed his boat and the army took Hugh and his Norwegian crew captive.

Hugh had the appearance of a crusty old seaman. He was tall, gaunt, and bony, and his only clothing was the captain's uniforms he had on board at the time of his capture. But his disposition more resembled that of Father Christmas. Grace Nash first met Hugh at Santo Tomas when her young sons mistook him for a pirate. He played along, and the boys were excited to meet a buccaneer. The game continued even as the boys realized the kind older man was not a genuine pirate. With Hugh, the children were no longer waiting in a chow line in a prison camp. They were in an imaginary world, on a ship prowling the high seas. They ran about at his command, hoisting invisible sails and preparing for battle against enemy pirate ships.

Hugh called the boys his "maties" or his "men." Grace thought it was her sons' greatest honor to be considered part of Hugh's crew. She watched with gratitude when they left the chow line with meager portions and Hugh told her boys a tale to stop them from crying. He'd point at the thin layer of mush and announce, "You think this is bad?" Then, he'd launch into one of his real-life stories of high-seas adventure, how he'd battled hurricane-strength winds or hungry sharks. Adults liked Hugh's stories as well. They packed into his evening lectures at Santo Tomas and listened with rapture as he described his marine escapades.

After he was transferred to Los Baños, Hugh turned his attention to Cobb. She likely envisioned making a life with him after the war. Hugh's adventurous spirit might have prompted him to follow Cobb on her next assignment—to San Diego, Annapolis, or Panama. His untimely death put an end to that dream.

Though Dorothy had never much cared for her chief nurse, she had always respected her. More than the younger nurse ever wanted to admit, Laura Cobb took responsibility for others' well-being. Cobb always positioned herself between the guards and her nurses. She hid their records, negotiated supplies, and absorbed their many crises. In this way, she was similar to the kindhearted captain.

It was Hugh's compassion, in fact, that eventually contributed to his death. About eight months earlier, he had given his last can of condensed milk to Grace Nash. Her baby was starving, and Hugh thought the infant needed it more than he did. Few inmates would have been so generous—it went against survival instincts. Prisoners bartered, traded, and stole. But few shared. All Hugh asked was for Grace to play "Danny Boy" for him at the next camp concert.

In the early stages of his illness, a liquid diet could have helped him. That he died in sacrifice did not take away the sting of his passing. Cobb remained next to her dear friend, who was covered in a sheet, until he was collected for burial. The camp carpenters constructed a coffin from scrap wood. And Grace Nash arranged for the camp orchestra to play his favorite song, "Danny Boy." The next day, the lyrics echoed in the inmates' minds as Hugh was laid to rest: "*'Tis you, 'tis you must go and I must bide.*"

———————

Dorothy had always been a hard sleeper. Even with the hardships of internment, the fatigue of a twelve-hour workday usually sent her into deep dream cycles. One time, nurse Peg had tried to rouse her after a pregnant prisoner went into labor. The nurses needed to take turns staying with the woman, and Dorothy was due for a shift. In her slumber, Dorothy mumbled nonsensically, "It's forbidden, she can't," as if Peg might go to the infirmary and tell the expecting mother her labor was postponed due to camp regulations. In the morning Dorothy told Peg how she'd had the funniest dream that someone was trying to wake her because a baby was on the way.

Now Dorothy was fast asleep as her roommate Eldene lay in bed, listening to truck engines rolling past the barracks. Eldene went to the window and crouched down, trying to determine the source of the sinister sound. She heard truck doors slam and the sound of soldiers' boots slogging through the mud. Dorothy still slept.

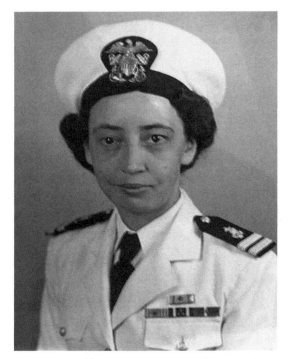

Navy nurse Eldene Paige. *Courtesy of Bureau of Medicine and Surgery*

"Dottie, wake up!" Eldene urged.

This time Dorothy responded, the sleepy fog vanishing as she joined Eldene by the window. They whispered concerns as to why a line of trucks had formed near the guards' barracks. They sensed something significant was happening, and they needed to know what. Though no one was allowed outside the barracks during the overnight hours, they decided to take the risk. If the guards were preparing for a mass execution, could they alert others? Might they be able to run toward the barbed wire and hide in the hills?

The women stood in front of their barrack with their backs to the wall, trying to fade into the darkness. They saw sentries removing shovels from the shed and placing them on the back of the truck. The women held their breath as adrenaline charged through their bodies. They feared that the Japanese army had ordered their Formosan guards to dig a mass grave. It was a rumor that had been rippling through the camp for weeks. The inmates knew that the Japanese army was obsessed with honor and loathed the indignity of surrender. With the Allied forces advancing, the threat of retribution was very real. The women backed into the barracks, uncertain what to do.

From their cubicle, Dorothy and Eldene listened as a guard addressed the barrack's hall monitor. To their amazement, they heard the guard indicate that the entire garrison was leaving Los Baños. The administrative committee was summoned to the commander's office for further instruction. The commander announced that he was turning the camp over to their control. He directed the men to the food stores and suggested the supply would last them two months if they were responsible. He also warned no one should leave the camp. The area was still under Japanese occupation.

The committee members contained their excitement as the commander addressed the paperwork he wanted to process prior to his departure. One inmate was enlisted to type up the names of the twenty-one hundred prisoners. The commander took the original and gave the carbon copy to the administrative committee. The commander also wanted a signed statement that on January 9, he turned the camp over to the committee's control.

The commander climbed into his sedan and followed the line of trucks through the front gate. The head of the administrative committee stood by the loudspeaker and waited until the last truck slipped from view. Then he spoke into the microphone, broadcasting the news: the Japanese had departed. He begged for order as inmates began to rush toward the guards' former barracks and push their way inside.

Some inmates had no inclination to loot the guards' former barracks, considering it a point of pride to say they did not care to own anything that had once belonged to a guard. But others were far too desperate to miss the opportunity. Weakened prisoners stripped the barracks clean of everything that had value. Buckets, tools, tables—anything the rubber-kneed inmates could lift. Inmates who hadn't sat in a proper seat for years eagerly dragged chairs back to their cubicles. Those with bug-ridden beds snatched sentries' mattresses and laboriously hauled them across campus. The looting paused only when a voice on the loudspeaker announced a flag-raising ceremony. No one wanted to miss that.

At sunrise, Dorothy and the other nurses joined a mass of people gathering near a flagpole that had been hastily constructed from bamboo. The inmates represented eleven countries. The majority were American, but there was also a sizable British population, and other inmates were Australian, Canadian, Dutch, Norwegian, Polish, and Italian. There were a handful of Filipinos, such as Basilia, one lone Nicaraguan, and a single Frenchman. None of the inmates expected to see their country's flag. Early in their captivity, the guards had rid the camp of any flags, patriotic music, or national symbols.

Or so they thought. The loudspeaker popped as the operator pointed the microphone toward a spinning record. Dorothy heard the white noise of the needle running on the outer rim. A horn blared one short note and then Bing Crosby's voice filled the camp with "The Star-Spangled Banner." Dorothy began to cry. The guards had never confiscated the record. They saw the famous actor's name and assumed it was music from one of his films.

The crowd gasped and then went quiet as an American flag ran up the bamboo pole. Parents lifted their children so they could glimpse the stars and the stripes for the first time. The nurses put their hands over their hearts and wept at the sight of a flag they had not seen since their capture at Santa Scholastica, when they had to watch it burn. Dorothy didn't know who in the camp had concealed an American flag for three years, but she was grateful to the person who had risked its safekeeping.

The flag was lowered, carefully removed, and returned to the owner. Great Britain's flag was hoisted next. A British internee had secreted the Union Jack for three years, and someone had hidden a record of the Royal Marine Band performing "God Save the King." It was the British inmates' turn to soak in the patriotism. All too soon, the flag was lowered. If the enemy returned, the administrative committee did not want retribution for flying an Allied flag. Some announcements closed the meeting. First and foremost: Los Baños had a new name—Camp Freedom. The inmates cheered.

The administrative committee announced new rules, and strongly cautioned inmates not to leave the camp while they awaited liberation. They were in a war zone and straying was a risk. Meals would be increased to thrice daily at full rations. In the interest of safety, a roll call would be conducted at night to ensure everyone was accounted for.

"Of course, it will no longer be necessary for you to bow during roll call," the announcer quipped. A few people smiled at each other. Others released an appreciative whoop. Their captors were gone, and freedom was near!

––––––––––––––

Within a day, the prisoners who were formerly radio operators applied their skills to the receivers the guards had left behind. They tuned into KGEI, a relatively new broadcast station in San Francisco capable of sending sound waves across the Pacific. Hearing President Roosevelt address the nation alleviated many fears. Japanese-run newspapers had long asserted that California had been bombed. Some of the guards had claimed Roosevelt had syphilis. Others swore he'd been pushed from office after the United States was conquered. And a visiting Japanese diplomat told inmates how the empire had seized the West Coast and fought their way to Chicago, where the Native Americans put up a great resistance. At the time, the inmates had muffled smirks about the Chicago comment. Now they knew for certain it was all lies. Their homeland was safe.

The next day, a voice on the loudspeaker urged inmates to stop what they were doing and listen. A radio operator held the microphone up to the receiver. A news bulletin detailed how General MacArthur had successfully led sixty-eight thousand men of the US Sixth Army into Lingayen Gulf, about 130 miles northwest of Manila. The battle of Luzon had begun! Subsequent reports confirmed that the war was getting closer to Los Baños. The Sixth Army was a mere two hundred miles away, with troop estimates as high as two hundred thousand men.

In the following days, inmates disregarded the advice to remain inside the gates. After months of starvation, they were motivated to forage for wild-growing foods. Threadbare locals arrived, eager to exchange fruits and vegetables for clothing. Dorothy rummaged through her trunk for her civilian dresses and traded them for bananas, papayas, mung beans, and vegetables. She kept only one dress, which she planned to wear home after liberation. The rest she was glad to be rid of. They reminded her of happier days.

Area civilians weren't the only ones interested in entering the camp. A guerrilla leader donated several water buffalo. Some prisoners thought he was just a caring local, but the warrior wanted information about the guards and their movements. Several young men in the camp gladly told the leader what they knew. The more food they consumed and the better they felt physically, the more they seethed with anger toward their former captors.

The majority of the camp focused on rebuilding their health. Inmates harvested syrup from the trees and added it to their morning rice to incorporate sugar back into their diet. Others took advantage of the coconuts that the locals delivered by handcart. The prisoners soon stared hungrily at the commander's prized bull. The administrative committee approved slaughtering the animal, as well as twenty pigs from the garrison's piggery. The inmates got their first taste of meat in months, but the anxious lines that formed outside the latrine reflected the inmates' inability to stomach a richer diet. Though the supply of food now seemed endless, the administrative committee didn't trust the situation. They arranged for all inmates to receive a small supply of rice to keep in their barracks in case of emergency.

———————

When trucks roared into camp on January 13, the inmates eagerly assumed their liberators had swiftly made their way from Luzon to Los Baños. But it wasn't a rescue. The entire Japanese garrison had returned, and Camp Freedom was no more. "We are here to protect you," Major Iwanaka assured the dejected inmates as he reassumed command.

Dorothy was sickened by the guards' return, and she had no sympathy for their fatigued, defeated appearance. She learned they'd been forced to dig trenches for the Japanese infantry. The officers felt demeaned for being handed a shovel and told to get to work, and once the job was done they were confused about what to do next. So they simply returned to the camp, and they came in with a fury. Konishi and the other officers were outraged to discover that inmates had looted their former barracks. Iwanaka had not expected the administrative committee to move into his office and was alarmed that several radios were missing. The commander was most upset at the loss of his favorite rice bowl, which had the Japanese imperial flag painted on the bottom. Why, he wondered, would someone disrespect him by taking his beautiful bowl?

The guards ransacked the inmates' barracks the next day to retrieve their personal belongings. The officers took inventory of the camp supply and then demanded that looted items be returned. Calls for the missing radio were repeated, and the threat of punishment increased. Then, in a surge of savagery, the sentries brutally beat a local whom they accused of coming too close to the camp's perimeter. The guards tied the young Filipino to a post and viciously attacked him in view of trembling inmates.

The Los Baños inmates were once again prisoners of an angry enemy facing defeat. The head counts intensified as Konishi sought retribution. The warrant officer cut rations down to a handful of rice every other day. The only other food he permitted was a type of cornmeal. It required husking, but the inmates did not know how to do it. Basilia demonstrated for her fellow nurses, and the women wondered if the caloric reward was even worth the effort. With the inmates fading, Konishi escalated efforts to exhaust them. Prisoners were forced to stand three times a day outside of their barrack and bow to their captors as a sign of respect. Within days, fragile inmates strained to bow and to remain standing during the count. For some, the issue was physical. But for others, the struggle was psychological.

Inmate John Howard Hell felt he'd had enough. During the brief period of Camp Freedom, he had begun leaving the grounds to gather fresh food for the camp—a godsend to the starving inmates. Now that the Japanese were back, such activity was again forbidden. But Howard was not going to let that stop him anymore.

As a young man, Howard had been fearless. Born in 1910, he grew up near the Ozarks in Rolla, Missouri. When carnivals came to town, the young Howard would volunteer to wrestle showmen who boasted they could take down any man in the crowd. Howard quickly pinned the professionals, and even when he met his match, he refused to concede until his opponent relinquished in fear of killing the young challenger.

Howard had first come to the Philippines as a mining engineer. He married his wife in June 1941, but because of new US restrictions on dependents in the Philippines, his wife had to remain in Missouri when he returned to his job as a superintendent at a gold mine. After the invasion, Howard eluded the Japanese in the mountains. His survival was uncertain, and Howard decided to give himself up when he saw a bulletin that promised repatriation to anyone who presented the document as they surrendered to Japanese soldiers. There was no limit, the bulletin promised, as to how many civilians could surrender under the same document. The bulletin was a trap, and Howard eventually ended up at Santo Tomas.

The man who was once fearless in a fight was crushed by the forced inactivity at the camp. Debilitated by anxiety, he grew a thick beard and went barefoot, a shadow of his former self. His friends told him he resembled a medieval painter's depiction of a saint. When he heard about the opportunity to work at Los Baños, he applied for transfer and was accepted.

His mental health improved at the new camp, and he took on the position of head gardener. Among the eggplants and the onions, Howard found his strength to fight. He couldn't brawl with the guards, but he could resist their efforts to starve the camp. Howard became the Robin Hood of the garrison's garden. He declared vegetables damaged and unfit for guard consumption so that he could give them to ailing prisoners, often single women with children. After the garrison abandoned the camp, Howard left each day and returned with fruit, vegetables, and meat for inmates who needed it most.

When the guards reassumed command, Konishi threatened fatal consequences for such excursions, posting a simple note that warned, "Will shoot after 3:30 PM Sunday." Howard ignored the threat. He was tired of death. The man who had once challenged professional wrestlers still had a bit of scrap left in him. On the Monday after the garrison returned, he pushed his way through the fencing, collected fruits and vegetables, and then walked casually back down the hill, reentering the camp without being apprehended by the guards. He did the same on Tuesday, carrying a dead chicken in one hand and a sack of coconuts and bananas in another. This time, a guard saw him slip back through the barbed wire, raised his rifle, and took aim. Three shots blasted across the camp. Howard was hit in the chest and head and fell to the ground, dead.

The camp raged. Howard had single-handedly prevented many inmates from developing beriberi, and there were prisoners who were alive because of him. When he was shot, he wasn't even escaping. He was *returning*. The members of the administrative committee planned a funeral for the next morning, but when they realized that the entire camp planned to attend, they feared a riot. They rescheduled the event for two hours earlier and informed only twenty of Howard's closest friends of the time change. Howard was buried in the drizzling rain. Flower wreaths were scattered onto his coffin, and then heavy shovels of mud filled the grave.

There were inmates who looked at Howard's grave and felt envy. Only the dead in Los Baños were finally free of their oppression. But others realized that a burial in the thick mud meant the body would never leave the camp. The prisoner's remains were sentenced to stay at Los Baños for all of eternity. The thought of such a punishment motivated many debilitated inmates to hold on to what was left of their fading lives.

16

Roll Out the Barrel

———————

HELEN GORZELANSKI HOVERED over patient charts. It was almost 7:00 AM and she needed to finalize her reports from the night shift. Dorothy joined Helen at the front desk and skimmed the reports, trying to gauge the day ahead. Wet beriberi patients were swollen and miserable. Dry beriberi patients were skeletal and wretched. Anemic inmates complained of thirst. And severely malnourished prisoners were on the brink of organ failure.

The crack of a rifle blast broke the women's concentration. Dorothy looked up at Helen. The detonation wasn't a truck backfiring—it sounded like a gunshot. Dorothy hesitantly suggested it sounded like it came from inside the camp. Had the guards shot another inmate? What was happening?

Dana tore through the lobby and burst out the front door. Dorothy and Helen rushed from the infirmary and saw the doctor sprinting toward the fence. An inmate was slumped on the ground, bleeding from his shoulder. Guards screamed at Dana and ordered him back with bayonet tips. Dana halted and assessed the man from a distance.

Dorothy recognized the wounded inmate as George J. Louis, an American in his late twenties who had been a Pan-Am mechanic. Blood poured from a wound just above his clavicle. It appeared the bullet had missed every major organ and artery. George would live, but he needed to be treated in the infirmary immediately.

George, like Howard Hell two weeks earlier, had left the camp to forage for food. George attempted to coordinate his return with the guards' daily calisthenics. Almost the entire garrison performed the routine each morning, except for the officers and the guards on duty in the guard towers. The sentries locked their weapons in a warehouse and then stripped down to loincloths and sandals. They lunged, jumped, and showed their strength to the deteriorating inmates. Most inmates stayed in their barracks, trying to conserve enough energy to stay standing during the morning roll call.

On the other side of the barbed wire, George heard the garrison begin their routine. He slid back into the camp and walked toward the barracks. A sentry in the guard tower saw him near the perimeter. He aimed at George and fired.

In the distance, Dorothy could not hear George crying and whimpering in pain. He writhed on the ground as an officer strode to the commander's office to report the incident. In the dim morning light, Dorothy saw the silhouettes of Dana and a few members of the administrative committee motioning frantically between the infirmary and the wounded man. After fifteen slow minutes, the old commander summoned the committee members to his office.

"Our doctor has pronounced him dead," Major Iwanaka said coldly. An interpreter translated the message as if he was repeating a supply order.

The committee members protested—George was not dead! He was crying, breathing, and conscious. The man needed medical treatment, which he was guaranteed under the Geneva Convention. One inmate rattled off the various articles within the Geneva Convention that mandated access to medical care. Iwanaka considered the new information. Very well, he told the interpreter. If the man is still alive, then he must be executed.

The inmates begged Iwanaka to spare George's life. They again cited the Geneva Convention and urged the commander to honor international law. Iwanaka was not convinced, and the interpreter repeated the commander's bizarre logic: On January 13, when the garrison returned to camp, guards were directed to shoot to kill any prisoner caught trying to escape. The guard had shot George but did not kill him. Therefore the order must be completed. The inmates argued against such nonsense, but after watching the desperate men implore his interpreter to intervene, Iwanaka stood up and walked away. For him, the issue was settled.

An emotional vein stretched through the camp, pumping fear into every barrack. Adults whispered about the wounded prisoner, trying to comprehend the impending violence. Would the guards actually shoot the man? Or might they relent once they sensed the entire camp had been sufficiently frightened into submission? The inmates fretted for the next ninety minutes. George remained by the fence, occasionally letting out a whimper or a slight movement. He was still alive, the inmates reassured each other.

And then guards surrounded George. The bleeding man moaned as several sentries heaved him onto a makeshift stretcher and carried him outside the barbed wire. Out of sight, the guards dumped George into a dense bamboo thicket. In the ward, Dorothy heard a single blast. The executioners then hauled the dead man back to the infirmary.

Dana and Dorothy stood alongside the stretcher. Dana wanted to document the murder. The body had to be lifted onto an examination table for an autopsy. Dorothy slid her hands under the back of George's head and prepared to lift her end. She felt his shattered skull and instinctively pulled her hands back. George's shredded cortex coated her fingertips. She couldn't stop herself from wincing.

Dorothy had seen so much as a nurse. At Cavite, she had administered morphine to men who'd violently lost a limb, with only frayed nerve endings protruding from the stump. She had comforted the dying sailor with the fully exposed torso oozing bowels. She examined rotted flesh, treated infections, and wiped pus that leaked from wet beriberi patients. But she had never handled brain matter, and now it felt as though she had truly touched death. She washed her hands, trying to scrub away the defeating sadness she felt from the execution.

Throughout the day, Dorothy contemplated why she was so unnerved by the brain matter. The brain, she concluded, was different. It held a person's thoughts and directed his dreams. The brain was the creator of sympathy and understanding. George's brain, the center of his being, was blown apart with a single blast. His hopes and dreams were mere remnants that smeared onto her skin.

The patients in Dorothy's ward did not need to know her trauma. She persevered through her shift, returning to the sink whenever her emotions returned. Each time, she let the water flow over her hands and hoped each rinsing would finally eliminate the sensation. She would learn in years to come that it never quite went away.

———————

On the morning George Louis was executed, 121 US Army Rangers invaded enemy territory in Luzon and stealthily advanced thirty miles to the prison camp near Cabanatuan. Aided by guerrilla forces, the rangers were on a mission to liberate the 513 prisoners, many of them survivors of the Bataan Death March, who had endured years of disease and slave labor. Almost twenty-seven hundred American military men had already died at Cabanatuan.* The survivors, now mere slivers

———————

* This number does not include the Filipino and American lives lost during the Bataan Death March, on the hell ships, or at Camp O'Donnell.

of skin and bone, had miraculously sidestepped the constant movement of prisoners out of the camp. Able-bodied men were constantly yanked from Cabanatuan and crammed onto the "hell ships" destined for slave labor camps in Japan.

American guerrilla Robert Lapham had hoped for years to liberate the camp. Lapham was once an army lieutenant assigned to an outpost that observed enemy movement. After the fall of Bataan, his major gave him the option to surrender or slip into the mountains and try to survive on his own. Lapham chose the mountains, and over the years he had built up a force of more than thirteen thousand guerrillas, most of them Filipino. His troops stalked Cabanatuan for years. Shadow figures lurked behind trees and then told of the random executions and daily beatings. They described mass graves filled with diseased corpses and emaciated men who looked ready to follow. Though Lapham burned to storm the camp and rescue the prisoners, the geography worked against him. The inmates would have to hike through the mountains to safety, and Lapham knew they were too debilitated to manage the escape. He settled for harassing the Japanese while waiting for US reinforcements to arrive.

In Lapham's monitoring of the camp, he knew all its movements and terrors. Based on the previous weeks' activities, he believed a mass execution was imminent. On January 26, he delivered a grave assessment to a US intelligence officer. The Sixth Army had to strike immediately. Otherwise, Lapham warned, the Cabanatuan inmates would be slaughtered before the month's end. Disturbed by Lapham's report, the intelligence officer convinced the Sixth Army's commanding general to begin planning that same day. Lieutenant Colonel Henry Mucci was selected to lead the stealth team, which would be joined by guerrilla captain Juan Pajota and two hundred of his warriors, many of them lacking firearms but ready for battle.

Mucci needed several days to organize the raid and position his troops within striking distance. On January 30, rangers and guerrillas surrounded the camp and crouched in a field waiting for the signal to attack. While the men crept into position, an aerial decoy flew low, directing the guards' focus to the sky. The pilot held the sentries' attention for at least twenty minutes as he circled back, played with the altitude, and then feigned a crash into the side of the mountain before reappearing moments later. With everyone in place and the guards distracted, the liberators unlocked their weapons and charged at the camp.

The first order of business was to kill every guard, which the rangers and guerrillas swiftly accomplished. The second task—convincing fearful prisoners that they were not going to die—proved a greater challenge. Terrified inmates heard gunfire and scattered into dark corners and muddy trenches. The most infirm lay in bed and begged the invaders for their lives. Others refused to leave. It was all a ploy, they believed, to trick them into slaughter. They didn't trust the Filipino guerrillas, and the American Army Rangers' uniforms and helmets were unfamiliar. The suspicious inmates feared the rangers were actually Germans posing as Americans. The rangers tried announcing the liberation, hoping their familiar American voices would resonate with the shaking prisoners.

"It's the Americans, get the hell out of here!" one ranger bellowed.

"Take it easy, fellows. The Yanks are here," another liberator tried to assure the prisoners.

Some of the inmates were convinced by the Texas twangs and New England accents. They followed the rangers through the broken barbed wire and joined the procession heading toward American lines. Others realized their rescue was underway and stumbled back to their barracks to collect their belongings.

None of these reactions were what the rangers had expected. In Europe, the Allied forces had begun liberating the Nazi death camps. Survivors stood cautiously near the barbed wire, mindful after years of beatings not to meet the rescuers' gaze. The Philippine liberations did not follow the same script, and the rangers were not prepared for the inmates' long-tortured nerves. The rescuers had assumed the prisoners would eagerly embrace freedom. To a certain extent, the prisoners had dreamed of doing just that, but the actual event was so startling that inmates flew into a self-preservation response.

The hesitant inmates quickly irritated the liberators. With thousands of Japanese soldiers lurking in the area, time was of the essence. Yet the distrusting prisoners wanted questions answered. Why is your uniform different than I remember? The United States really switched helmet styles? What is a "ranger"? Are you *actually* from California? The rangers resorted to dragging the hesitant men from the camp. On the other side of the barbed wire, the most fragile inmates were organized onto the backs of water buffalo or stretchers carried by guerrillas.

Days later, the Sixth Army swept through the camp. They pulled back floorboards and cut open mattresses to collect whatever secret documents the inmates had managed to maintain during their ordeal. Journals, logs, and letters stood as witness to the atrocities the prisoners had endured. The US Armed Forces were planning on a victory in Europe and the South Pacific. And when their enemy surrendered, they wanted justice. The Geneva Convention, despite the Japanese Imperial Army's dismissals, would not be ignored.

In the coming days, the US military quickly learned that Americans loved liberation stories. Every major newspaper ran daily reports about the raid, the heroes, and the newly freed prisoners. Reporters interviewed exuberant families who heard their missing son or husband was finally coming home. Photographers snapped a picture of Mucci's wife, Marion, beaming with pride for her husband's heroics.

The smaller newspapers picked the stories off the wire, bringing the Cabanatuan raid to even the remotest parts of the country.

The raid felt like a significant war victory, as much as any major land battle or successful marine attack, but Americans wanted more. The day after the liberation at Cabanatuan, news stories alerted readers to other camps in the Philippines where both military personnel and civilians were in dire need of rescue. The reports also assured readers that the Cabanatuan survivors were doing well "and already looked like new men." The exaggeration was part of the odd insulation the newspapers wrapped around the prison camps. Atrocities against the deceased, particularly those on the Bataan Death March, were articulated by survivors. But editors added a feel-good element to the story, often focusing on the rangers' heroic efforts or the prisoners' gratitude for liberty. Men were described as devouring several hamburgers in one sitting and enjoying the feel of shoe leather on their feet for the first time in years. By and large, the stories spared readers from the atrocities the army was just beginning to fully comprehend.

The stunning realization surfaced on the march back to Allied territory. The near-naked prisoners resembled skeletons. Most did the "Cabanatuan Shuffle," hobbling to spare themselves from putting full pressure on the inflamed nerves in their feet. Jerry Steward, husband of nurse Basilia Torres Steward, was among the procession of pained prisoners. Jerry had been transferred to Cabanatuan from Bilibid Prison in October 1943. His health spiraled at the second camp, and he now weighed 114 pounds less than when the war began. His shrapnel wounds still bothered him, particularly in one of his legs. But he walked the distance to American lines, eager to see if he could get back to Manila and find his wife.

Other men were also committed to enduring the painful walk to freedom. They wanted the dignity that came from managing on their own. The rangers, however, were astonished by the prisoners' ailments. A few were amputees. Many were missing teeth or chunks of their lice-infested hair. Most suffered night blindness from malnutrition. With few exceptions, almost every man weighed less than a hundred pounds. They strongly resembled the prisoners who had been liberated from Auschwitz just days earlier. The US Army surmised that the other Japanese prison camps were likely just as inhumane as Cabanatuan had been.

Bilibid Prison, just south of Manila, was of great concern to military leaders, as was the camp at Santo Tomas. Because the army was advancing toward Manila, the crisis in these two camps would soon be resolved. But the twenty-one hundred inmates at Los Baños, situated as it was in the mountains and not en route to Manila, would have to remain imprisoned for now.

At Santo Tomas, as many as four inmates were dying each day from starvation. A registered nurse working at the infirmary confided in her diary how she could tell from appearance which inmates would be next. She described on February 1 how the guards slaughtered a water buffalo in front of starving inmates, who pleaded for a shred of meat. The sentries allowed the inmates to fight over the blood, entrails, and ears they left behind. Those who couldn't secure a scrap left in defeat.

The Santo Tomas inmates encouraged each other to hold on. Liberating forces were near—they could feel it. The ground quaked from bomb concussions and their noses burned from the explosives. On February 3, inmates received further assurance after an American plane flew low and the pilot's goggles plummeted into the camp with an attached note: "Roll out the barrel, Christmas will be either today or tomorrow!"

The inmates tried to anticipate just when deliverance would come and what it would be like. They did not have long to wonder. After sunset that same day, tanks crashed through the main gate and rumbled up to the main building. As at Cabanatuan, fearful inmates fled from what they assumed were Germans intending to deceive them. Others were convinced by the colloquial nicknames, such as "the Georgia Peach," that the soldiers had painted on the sides of the armored vehicles.

Santo Tomas was a liberation in stages. The guards retreated to the education building and hid behind two hundred hostages. The hostages were held at bayonet point while the US Army shelled the building. Across the camp, newly freed inmates celebrated their freedom.

Even after the camp was finally rid of the Japanese guards two days later, the inmates realized they were not yet fully free. They had to remain inside the prison until Manila was completely under Allied control. The enemy still occupied the northern parts of the city, but it was anticipated that their retreat would be quiet and quick. In the coming weeks, however, the Japanese soldiers sprang into a banzai charge. If the Allied forces were going to win the capital, then the Japanese Imperial Army would ensure they won nothing but destruction.

Steams of civilians fled the northern parts of the city as US and Filipino forces launched into urban combat. By the end of the battle, the fighting had destroyed the city and the Japanese army had killed more than one hundred thousand civilians. The US Army was astounded by the brutality. The Japanese soldiers inflicted upon Manila the same type of destruction as they'd wreaked upon Nanking in 1937. Allied soldiers unearthed bodies of beaten men with their hands tied behind their back. In a Red Cross building, they found charred patients who'd been strapped to their beds and then burned to death. All through the city, soldiers stumbled on the corpses of naked women who were raped before they were stabbed repeatedly with a bayonet. The bodies of children and infants were discovered in apartments, churches, and schools. There was no mercy for even Manila's smallest citizens.

17

Today We Either Live or Die

DOROTHY STUMBLED THROUGH the ward. A patient watched as she tried to steady herself on weak legs. She offered a reassuring smile and joked how she walked like a "drunken sailor." The patient had heard the quip before—other nurses made light of their failing bodies. They tried to laugh when they gripped the stair railing and ascended one step at a time, pausing between movements like an elderly woman. And they tried self-deprecating humor whenever they tumbled in front of patients, wisecracking that they really needed to stop drinking before their shift.

Chief Nurse Cobb encouraged her nurses to continue on. The end was near, she assured them. But the women were not convinced. Konishi halted rations, and the nurses depleted their emergency rice stores. They were reduced to eating swamp weeds. The women wondered if the army even knew about Los Baños. Each time they raised the question, Cobb repeated her assurance that help was on the way. "They are doing all they can," she promised.

It had been almost six weeks since Cobb had lost her friend Hugh. Dorothy noticed she no longer tried to pluck her gray hairs. Nor did she seem to notice when the coarser grays escaped her hairpins. Cobb had typically maintained a tidy appearance, and Dorothy sensed her stoic chief nurse was quietly fading. The twelve women were all declining, and they no longer resembled the group that had served together at Cavite. They had been playful then, shrieking with laughter over the dungarees and humoring each other by modeling the poorly fitting pants. Now it seemed like the only time they smiled was when they were trying to feign cheerfulness for the patients.

The women also noticed they no longer had energy to argue. The scorching disagreement between Helen and Dorothy in the autumn of 1943 about the orderlies seemed as though it had occurred among different versions of themselves. If the same scenario played out in February 1945, each woman would have shrugged and walked away. Neither had the physical strength or the mental capacity to expend on bickering. Death was all around them, and they felt their own was imminent.

Dorothy sat with patients as they passed from the world. She watched as each breath became separated by a lengthy pause. Ten seconds would pass between inhalations. Then fifteen. Twenty. *Lucky you*, Dorothy thought enviously when the breaths ceased. *May you rest in peace.*

One night, Dorothy thought she had died in her sleep. She woke to the realization she was not breathing and she did not feel the beating of her own heart. She felt relief to think her misery was over, but then she reflexively took a breath and sadly acknowledged she was still alive. Dorothy was not opposed to a peaceful passing, especially as rumors of mass execution loomed.

The inmates feared the Japanese would slaughter the entire camp. And on February 22, they watched with trepidation as the guards set up machine guns at various points around the perimeter and then turned the barrels inward. One prisoner told Mary Rose that she should play dead in the event of a mass shooting. That way, the inmate suggested helpfully, the guards would think they'd already killed her. Others plotted which direction they should run or whether it was possible to hide until the massacre was over and the garrison abandoned the camp.

Chief Nurse Cobb knew of the rumors. Concerning, she agreed, but no excuse to break rank. The women were to adhere to their schedule as planned. Dorothy and Peg Nash were scheduled for the night shift and she expected them to appear on time. Dorothy reported for duty, not certain if she would be alive in the morning.

Dorothy did not know that others were getting into position as well. In Manila, members of the 11th Airborne's B Company were preparing to sleep on the tarmac so that they would be ready to fly at dawn. Across the lake, the 672nd Amphibian Tractor Battalion Division loaded into fifty amtracs* and crossed the lagoon in the black night, using only compasses to guide them through the inky water. And in the woods surrounding Los Baños, Filipino guerrillas and American reconnaissance troops crept into position.

———————

Death was so common that the infirmary staff filled out death certificates in advance for declining patients, adding the time of death and final information once the act was complete. At the other end of the spectrum, late February brought new life to the hospital with the birth of two baby girls. Each was underweight, and their emaciated mothers did not have breast milk to feed their babies. The infirmary staff fed the newborns water sprinkled with powdered milk. Dorothy sadly thought the babies resembled plucked chickens.

———————

* An amtrac, or amphibious tractor, was a flat-bottomed military vehicle on tracks, able to move on land or across water.

The newborns brought a momentary happiness to the hospital. Death and decay dominated, yet the girls' mothers had somehow been able to conceive and bring their pregnancies to term. Their births felt like miracles, and the nurses were happy to hear the weak cries after each girl entered the world. But an upsetting mishap punctured the joy. One of the nurses inadvertently scalded one of the babies with a water bottle. It was an unforeseeable accident in which no one was to blame except for the captors. The water bottle wasn't very hot, and it was insulated by a blanket. But the newborn was so malnourished that her damaged skin burned on contact. The nurse involved was devastated, and the other women felt heartbroken. The injury slapped them with a reminder that any happiness was fleeting in the cruel camp.

Dorothy's night shift was almost over, and the rising sun reminded her to check on the little burn victim before the next nurse came on duty. Dorothy cooed as she brought the baby from the ward. Using a sweet voice, she marveled at how the little one still resembled a chicken who needed fattening. Dorothy changed the makeshift diaper, saving the cloth to be rinsed and reused. Then she fed the baby a watery milk substitute, patted her little back until she burped, and put her back in her bed.

It was not yet 7:00 AM as Dorothy began to update the patient charts. Outside the infirmary, she heard the garrison commence their morning calisthenics. They lunged and shadowboxed across the field in a exercise routine the inmates simultaneously resented and found ridiculous. An orderly watched from the window and joked he wasn't impressed. Dorothy agreed she could do the same exercises if she just had something to eat.

The sound of airplanes silenced them. The roar and deep vibration came from the north. It was the signal for ground troops to begin firing. Dorothy's eyes widened as she listened to the distinct rattling of machine gun fire. *Mass execution*, she thought. *They are killing us.* Dorothy ran into the ward and snatched the baby from her crib. She crouched by the front door and craned her neck to see what was happening outside. Ballooned parachutes swayed toward the ground. Peg Nash went to the window and saw the firefight.

Dear God, Peg thought. *Today we either live or die, but at least this suffering is going to be over.*

The ground forces burst into the camp. They'd been ordered not to take prisoners. The American soldiers took quick aim at the guard tower while the guerrillas charged with machetes at the near-naked sentries. Several guards ran toward the storage unit where their rifles were secured, fumbled with the lock, and were hacked to death trying to access their weapons. Others, including Konishi and Major Iwanaka, slipped through the barbed wire and headed into the dense woods.

Inmates outside their barracks ran for shelter, diving under beds and lying flat on the floor. The firefight that followed in the next fifteen minutes struck many as unreal, which produced strange behaviors. One young man ate a bowl of gruel under his bed. Two sisters hustled to the bathroom to brush their teeth so that they might seem attractive to their liberators. Dorothy, however, felt the realness of the battle. She was a war nurse.

Dorothy clutched the baby and exchanged alarmed glances with the orderlies. It was finally happening—just not how and when the inmates had expected. Like the rescue at Cabanatuan, the Los Baños inmates were still in enemy territory. The US Army intended to bring prisoners to a staging area two miles away at Laguna de Bay. From there, an amtrac would take them a short distance across the water. At the second staging area, inmates would be transferred into ambulances or trucks and driven to Bilibid Prison, which was now in Allied control.

The amtracs were massive, with open cargo holds that allowed for the transport of people or goods. The vehicle was lightly armored and moved briskly on land, but it was as slow as a water buffalo in water, moving at an unhurried five miles per hour. The army expected the water transfer to take several hours and require two trips between the staging areas.

A line of more than fifty amtrac vehicles trampled the fencing and rolled through the camp. One stopped in the infirmary's circular drive and American soldiers popped over the side and bounded into the building. Dorothy was stunned by their size. These men were mammoth. Only a few of the men in her camp weighed more than 120 pounds. The liberators seemed so tall and hefty. Conversely, the soldiers were shocked to see the size of the inmates. One soldier walked into a men's barrack and felt depressed to see the men's protruding rib cages. In his mind, he wondered, *What did they do to you?*

Chief Nurse Cobb hurried into the infirmary and began coordinating the patients' transfer to the beach. She had at least 150 patients who required special transport. A soldier listened to Cobb discuss the evacuation with his battalion leader, and his eyes drifted around the infirmary and rested on Dorothy.

"Ma'am, what are you holding?" he asked.

Dorothy looked at the blanket in her arms and realized she was still holding the baby. She raised the bundle to show the soldier. There was a moment of confusion as the soldier thought she was passing him the newborn. He took the bundle and the evacuation momentarily paused as the other soldiers teased the large man for cradling a baby. Dorothy laughed as she carried the little one back to her mother.

Peg approached one of the soldiers. "Do you have anything to eat?" she asked. He gave her a chocolate bar. Peg immediately ate half of it. Out of habit, she wrapped the remainder and saved it in her pocket, thinking she might need it in the future.

Dorothy passed out chocolate bars and cigarettes while Cobb conferred with Dana and the soldiers. Cobb had two nurses, she told the men, who were too sick to walk. They needed to be driven to the beach with the other immobile inmates. The ailing nurses,

Peg and Susie, were each given one of the infants to transport. They readily agreed, but then were surprised when they saw the bizarre, open-air vehicle intended to whisk them to the staging area. None of the women had ever seen a Jeep.

The Jeep sped to safety, but the troops of the 11th Airborne were having difficulty getting the other inmates onto the amtracs. People were *packing*. After years of imprisonment, the inmates' survival instinct made them want to pack up utensils, clothes, cooking gear, tins, and mementos. They did not know what was on the other side of that lagoon, and they felt compelled to prepare for continued deprivation. A few dug in their heels and insisted that the US Army feed them breakfast before they left.

Prisoners of war, the army continued to learn, were difficult to predict. Inmates long dreamed about liberation, but they were traumatized by years of terror. The sounds of machine gun fire and amtracs crashing into the camp elicited a mentality the liberation planners did not anticipate. They more likely expected inmates would cheer their saviors and then quickly and agreeably evacuate as instructed. Instead, the Los Baños inmates were packing their belongings and demanding a snack for the road.

"Get moving! Get moving!" the soldiers ordered.

Soldiers used military lingo to try and motivate the prisoners to move. One soldier told a nun that he would smoke her butt if she didn't get hopping. The nun dismissed the disrespectful young man and returned to packing her gear. The soldier likely felt both humiliated and amused by the failure.

There was no time to indulge the inmates. The army estimated the Japanese could strike within hours. They needed everyone to board the amtracs at once. Paratroopers yelled into barracks for an all clear, then they lit the buildings on fire. One soldier looked sadly at a toy box and the little stuffed giraffes on top. As he doused the barrack, he wondered how any army could imprison and starve children.

From the infirmary, Dorothy saw black smoke streaming from the barracks. She rushed outside to collect her own belongings and felt devastated to see her smoldering cubicle. Everything she owned was devoured by flames—the dress she'd planned to wear out of the camp, the letter from her parents, the sliver of soap. She was saving that soap! Most importantly, the sketch pad with caricatures of the nurses. It was from another lifetime at Cavite, when she had purchased the pad thinking she might learn how to draw. Uninspired by her own attempts, she had let the camp's dentist create funny pictures of the infirmary staff. There was nothing more important than that pad. Dorothy sat dejected on the infirmary stairs. She suddenly didn't care anymore about living.

The US Army had planned a brisk hour to load the freed prisoners and transport them to the beach. Maintaining the timetable was critical. The guerrillas estimated there were eight thousand Japanese soldiers stationed within a few hours' march. About fifteen hundred inmates were herded onto the amtracs, and the long line rumbled toward the beach.

The administrative committee told the rescuers to not forget about the clergy and missionaries who had been brought to the camp. The religious workers were latecomers to Los Baños, and the sentries initially segregated them in a different part of the camp. The officer in charge sent up an amtrac, likely regretting that the one chosen for the journey had been christened the "Impatient Virgin." Was the "Typhoon Tess" not available? Or the "Little Joe"?

The stragglers had to walk the two miles. Several of the nurses set out with a pushcart, trying with weakened legs to shove the cart to the beach. One of the carts lost a wheel, and the women were amazed when two guerrillas offered to carry the contents for the remainder of the journey. The nurses hadn't seen such brawn in years.

Thomas found Dorothy in front of the infirmary. He was also in a sour mood. He had intended to use a pushcart to haul his belongings to the staging area, but the cart went up in flames in the camp kitchen. Now he had to carry his suitcases. Two other remaining nurses, Eldene and Bertha, likely looked at Thomas with envy. At least he'd had time to gather his personal items. All Bertha had was a tin of brown sugar.

The major in charge of the liquidation demanded the attention of the group that was about to set out from the camp on foot. The beach was a two-mile walk, he explained. There were Japanese snipers in the trees, so the inmates needed to stay together. Dorothy, Eldene, Bertha, Thomas, and another man set out together. As they trudged from the camp, a swarm of guerrillas packed around them. Dorothy noticed how the guerrillas quietly scanned the trees and reacted to any disturbance. She felt reassured. These hills were their home, and they knew exactly how the land should look and sound.

The procession came upon a dead guard as they progressed from the camp. The major was unnerved that the sentry had gotten so far before he perished. They had to assume there were others in the area. The major implored the inmates to walk as fast as possible. Thomas looked down at the guard as he passed. He recognized the dead man. He had once put down his rifle and helped Thomas carry a bag of rice. Thomas whispered to Dorothy that he wished it were Konishi lying on the ground, not a benign guard who had helped struggling inmates.

The guerrillas became more confident as the convoy neared the beach. They began to sing the Philippine national anthem in Tagalog and then English.

"Buried already is the darkness of yesterday's suffering," they sang.

Bertha listened to the soft singing. She was in awe of the warriors. They had resisted the occupation, and they were now risking their lives to save the prisoners from certain death. As they arrived at the beach, Bertha felt the weight of the tin and realized she no longer needed the brown sugar. She was on the verge of freedom. She passed the tin to one of the guerrillas.

The amtracs disappeared in waves. Peg and Susie departed with the first transport. Mary Rose and her fiancé, Page, followed, each clutching several cans of corned beef. Dorothy, Eldene, and Bertha were among the last to arrive at the staging area. Dorothy sat under a coconut tree and removed her shoes. It would take several hours for the amtracs to return and she was exhausted. Bertha chatted with one of the paratroopers, asking him about the current events in the United States.

Dorothy nodded off, and when she awoke, the paratroopers were no longer entertaining the prisoners with news from home. They had formed an arc on the beach, facing into the jungle with their weapons ready. Dorothy heard gunfire in the distance. The Japanese soldiers were indeed coming for them. A diversionary force blocked the initial response from the enemy. But the battalion leader did not think they could hold the beach for long. Across the bay, they could see the amtracs making their way back toward the staging area.

As the amtracs began to reach the beach, the major ordered the remaining inmates and soldiers to board immediately. *Everybody out!* Dorothy approached the first amtrac in line and asked the men sitting up front if she had permission to board. The soldiers nodded at the women's nursing pins and wanted to know if they were military.

"Navy Nurse Corps," Dorothy confirmed.

The soldiers invited Dorothy and Eldene to stay atop the amtrac, where a breeze made the air feel cooler, instead of crowding into the hold. The vehicle pulled away, and Dorothy looked back at the beach and watched the staging area recede from view. More than three years earlier, she had stood above deck on the patrol torpedo boat drinking in the smoldering ruins of Cavite. She'd never anticipated becoming a prisoner of war. It didn't seem possible at the time. Now it felt as though her agonizing journey was finally coming to an end.

Dorothy's thoughts were interrupted. One of the inmates fainted in the hold. Dorothy directed the soldiers to lift him. She and Eldene situated the patient so he was under the shade of an umbrella and resting comfortably in Dorothy's arms. Dorothy recognized the young man as a frequent patient at the hospital. He was emaciated, and the walk to the beach had been more than his body could handle. He gasped awake and then fell back into Dorothy's arms for the remainder of the crossing.

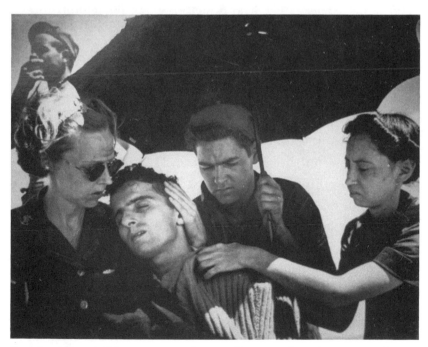

Dorothy Still and Eldene Paige tend to an ill inmate aboard an amtrac during the liberation of Los Baños. *Courtesy of Bureau of Medicine and Surgery*

Elsewhere, the other navy nurses were also still tending to their patients. Peg and Susie continued to carry the newborn girls. Others cared for the handful of inmates and soldiers who had been grazed by bullets. There was also a badly burned man who had run into the flames to rescue his belongings. Dorothy Still and the other eleven anchors were nursing until the end.

In the coming days, Konishi's plan for mass murder at Los Baños was redirected onto the civilian population. He ordered "guerrilla subjugation," a term the Japanese officers later claimed meant the interrogation of alleged guerrillas as well as civilians suspected of supplying food or information to enemy forces. But survivors later testified that subjugation was not a methodical or thoughtful process. Soldiers executed anyone caught in their crosshairs.

Konishi wanted revenge. He had seen guerrillas storming his camp with machetes, and he was certain it was local men who had hacked his sentries to death. One guerrilla's wife heard of the coming threat and tried to warn the area residents to evacuate. Many were confused or unconcerned and remained at home. Hundreds took shelter in a church, thinking the Japanese soldiers would respect the sacred edifice. In the church, the soldiers savagely stabbed and decapitated men, women, and children. They'd been ordered not to waste ammunition on "subjugation."

The same scenario repeated in the nearby town of Bai, where thirty Filipinos were shot in a coconut field. North of Bai, six hundred Chinese men, women, and children were tied together in groups of five and marched to a shallow trench. A menacing line of soldiers stood behind the victims. On cue, they stabbed the civilians until their lifeless bodies fell into the trench. Within days, the Japanese had massacred more than twelve hundred people.

Not all Japanese soldiers relished the annihilation. Each battalion included men who covered their eyes so they did not have to witness the slaughter. Some soldiers intentionally gave their intended victims time to flee. Some shot over their victims' heads or purposefully walked past trembling children and pretended the area was clear. But each battalion also included officers and soldiers who viewed the directive as undeniable, even if they disagreed with it. One company commander expressed doubts when he was ordered to massacre locals near Bai. The area residents had once shared hens and eggs with him. Still, he acquiesced; an order was an order.

18

Don't Worry Anymore About Me

THE AMTRAC RAMP fell forward with a thunk into the grass at the second staging area. Soldiers rushed to the vehicle to ease evacuees down the slope and toward a line of waiting trucks, helping them to step carefully through the mud and dodge the deep tire tracks made by previous caravans. As the later amtracs in the wave began to arrive, the freed inmates who'd been among the last to escape shared chilling stories of Japanese soldiers storming the beach. They were at a safe distance when the enemy pushed through, but they felt as though they'd made it by mere minutes.

The signal corps set up a camera to film the inmates in transit. An evacuee wearing only a bathrobe waved brightly at the camera. Others seemed oblivious as they struggled to climb into the open-air trucks. One middle-aged man tried to grab onto the side railing but didn't have the strength to heave himself over. A soldier had to push on the older man's bottom, as if he were a parent helping lift a child.

The cameras lingered on the survivors' emaciated figures, capturing a sense of the physical indignities they had faced. There were quiet indignities, however, that the cameras could not record. Numb evacuees stood on the field and realized they owned nothing. Some possessed only the clothes on their back. Their homes, businesses, material goods—everything was gone, and now they were on the verge of returning to a ruined life. Men with families in the Philippines were desperate to know whether their wives and children had survived the battle of Manila. And people with families in the States were anxious to let their loved ones know they were finally free and coming home.

For Dorothy, the dream of liberation had transpired alongside the long-dreaded reality of losing Thomas. One of Thomas's friends had wrangled passage for him to an American airfield, where he could fly directly home on a cargo plane. Everyone else was headed to Bilibid Prison. The rest of the journey home would take the rescued civilians weeks or months, depending on where they were headed.

Thomas couldn't wait to see his wife and children. He hurried toward the truck that would take him to the airfield. Dorothy went with Eldene and their patient onto a truck bound for Bilibid. There was no farewell or parting embrace. The friendship that had sustained Dorothy for almost two years ended without even a good-bye. Dorothy rode in the rumbling truck, feeling waves of exhaustion and pain that stretched through the long day.

It was after 5:00 PM when the motorcade finally approached Bilibid. The prison seemed downright palatial to the Los Baños inmates. Bilibid indeed resembled a castle, with two round gatehouses framing the front entrance and a large, open-air plaza inside the fortress wall. Dorothy wandered into the plaza, found a bench, and fell asleep. Except for a short nap, she had been awake and on duty for almost twenty-four hours.

Nurse Goldia O'Haver shook Dorothy awake. The Red Cross was distributing mail from the United States. Months-old mail, of course, but mail nevertheless. Dorothy looked around the courtyard. In a moment reminiscent of Santo Tomas, everyone was standing in some sort of line. Some queued at registration tables to have their names checked off logbooks. There was a line to pick up mail from the Red Cross as well as tables where evacuees could write letters home. Dorothy retrieved a letter from her mother, and then sat at one of the writing stations, pausing for a moment to admire the stacks of stationery and envelopes and piles of stubby pencils. Dorothy was amazed by the abundance—it had been more than three years since she had seen that many pencils. Dorothy wrote a letter to her parents. "Don't worry anymore about me," she urged. She cheerfully told them how wonderful it was to have American candy, cigarettes, and food once again.

The food, to Dorothy and the other former inmates, seemed to be in copious supply. The army had set out huge vats of a light bean soup, selected with the intent of reintroducing food slowly. Evacuees went through the line with a bowl shaped like a frying pan, into which a kitchen worker ladled a shallow serving. Many returned for a second or third helping. Some stared sadly at soldiers until they offered meat tins or fruit cups from their rations, while others unflinchingly rummaged through the garbage and claimed unopened cans of Spam that picky soldiers had tossed from their supper boxes. Dorothy was also amazed to see perfectly edible pork discarded. Who, she wondered, would throw out meat?

Empty five-gallon tin cans sent a cascade of evacuees hurrying toward the garbage. Those standing in the chow line saw the kitchen crew discarding the tins and immediately hustled toward them. Others instinctively followed, certain there was good reason for the excitement. The few who scored a can were delighted—five-gallon cans were ideal for washing laundry! The can could also store newly acquired belongings, such as the little pencils that disappeared from the Red Cross table.

Many of the American soldiers found the scene depressing. Grown adults shone with glee when handed a fruit cup. Children shook with jubilation when given a chocolate bar. These people had been gutted by deprivation. They were aching skeletons. General MacArthur saw some of the victims for himself when he toured both a military and a civilian prison camp. These were not internees, he concluded. They were concentration camp survivors.

The signal corps' cameras documented the emaciated men whose loose pants were belted high above their waists. They filmed the young women smiling at soldiers, and the children biting happily into chocolate bars. The footage was used to inspire Americans to support the war financially and to continue to believe in the fight. The cameras turned away, however, from the most upsetting sights, such as people openly weeping throughout the plaza. Some cried tears of relief at being given a hot meal, while others broke down after receiving painful news about their loved ones.

Letters from home told of beloved family members' deaths or terminal illnesses. News from soldiers or other evacuees revealed what had happened to servicemen they knew. Margaret Sherk was approached by a family friend with information about her husband, Bob. Margaret had planned on divorcing him after the war to marry fellow survivor Gerald Sams, the father of her second child. She learned that a divorce would not be necessary. Bob had died on a "hell ship" bound for Japan. His older brother John had perished on the same ship, and Bob watched as other inmates heaved John's body into the ocean. Within a few days, Bob succumbed to disease and was buried at sea. The Sherk family would one day put a headstone in a California cemetery to commemorate the brothers who had only each other in the end.

Elsewhere in the plaza, Grace Nash whispered with an intelligence corps officer and learned about the pressing reason for the rescue.

Headquarters had learned that the guards intended to massacre the inmates on February 23, probably either during the morning roll call or in the afternoon when retreating Japanese troops were scheduled to pass through the area. Grace lay awake that night, haunted by the officer's revelations. She had known a violent end was a possibility; all the inmates had. But to realize she survived her execution day sent waves of sleep-interrupting adrenaline through her body.

Many other evacuees were restless that night, particularly those who suffered cramps and nausea from overeating. The prison hospital received gorged patients seeking relief. There were also more than a hundred gravely ill evacuees as well as incoming casualties from area battles. Recognizing help was needed, Chief Nurse Cobb organized a schedule and put her nurses on shifts. The navy women dutifully reported for work, each one realizing during her first shift how much patient care had changed in the previous three years.

December 1941 had marked the nurses' last contact with the larger world and the date on which their medical knowledge paused. In the time they were locked away, the United States began utilizing penicillin. The navy nurses were fascinated by the development and asked the army physicians a plethora of questions. They wondered to themselves how much suffering could have been prevented had the antibiotic been available in the camps.

The nurses also learned new treatments for burns, a lesson that no doubt took them back to the bombing at Cavite, when screaming patients were brought into the wards with charred skin. At Cavite, the nurses had also been ordered to reuse syringes between patients without sterilizing. Now the army had single-use needles and pre-sterilized tubing for IVs. So much had changed, including the navy nurses themselves. For years, these women washed pus and blood from bandages, hung them in the sun to dry, and then reused them on other patients. Now they winced to see needles and other disposables in the trash. In their minds, all those items could be sanitized and reused—except that new regulations forbade recycling supplies. Military medicine had evolved, and the nurses were woefully out of date.

At the same time as they were catching up on their medical knowledge, they were working on adding to their weight. Peg Nash had left the camp at a gaunt sixty-eight pounds, and the other women were not much heavier. The nurses each gained between seven and ten pounds during their first week of freedom. Cobb, never one to carry extra weight, was thirty-five pounds lighter than she'd been before the war, but she knew that weight loss was not their only problem. They were all in need of restorative care, and Cobb pressed the army to release her nurses back to the United States for medical leave.

The hospital staff at Bilibid were disappointed. They were hoping the navy nurses would remain despite their ailments. Cobb stood firm, using her terse but quiet voice to let the army know her decision was final. The men acquiesced and began making arrangements to transfer them after army replacements arrived. Until then, the twelve ailing anchors were expected to maintain rank and deliver care to others, even though they so badly needed it themselves.

Jerry Steward tore through Bilibid looking for his wife, Basilia. He had been free for almost a month, having finagled his way into Santo Tomas after it was liberated in early February. He was disappointed when he arrived there and learned that his wife had been transferred to Los Baños, a camp he never knew existed. There was no way to get to her. He waited weeks for Basilia, rejecting any offer to leave the Philippines and return to Texas. He wanted to see his wife.

At last, Jerry found his wife safely among the navy nurses at Bilibid. The two embraced and then fussed over each other. They had been apart for almost three years and almost didn't recognize each other. Jerry stood at a soaring six feet four inches but was reduced to a slight

148 pounds. Basilia was a gaunt 82 pounds. It was no matter. They were finally together, and they did not want to be separated again.

Basilia and Jerry had much to tell each other. Most of it was not pleasant, but Jerry did have some good news. He had been promoted to the rank of captain and given the venerable Navy Cross for his bravery at Cavite. He was the most decorated engineer in the navy. The couple likely hoped his status would allow them to travel home together.

Within a few days, Basilia and Jerry learned they could indeed return to Texas together. Jerry was permitted to join the twelve nurses as they left Bilibid for Manila. The couple were allowed to be together—until the news photographers appeared and Jerry was asked to step out of view. The women were pushed into a staged photo upon arriving in Manila. They were briefly housed at Santo Tomas, a place they had hoped to never see again. Then, they flew south and east to the Philippine island of Leyte, where Admiral Thomas C. Kinkaid greeted them at his headquarters.

The nurses needed to rest, but first they were positioned outside Kinkaid's tent to pose for the news corps' cameras. They obediently surrounded the admiral and formed two lines. Peg smiled for the camera, but the rest ignored the photographers and chatted with each other.

The women were a raggedy, diseased group, and on instinct they packed tightly together. Edwina was still unwell from the mysterious illness that had first appeared back at Santo Tomas. Susie continued to smoke despite her emphysema. Chief Nurse Cobb—unbeknownst to her nurses—was coping with arthritis and a heart condition. Peg suffered from tuberculosis, which had yet to be diagnosed. And Dorothy was not feeling well. Like most of the other nurses, she was recovering from dry beriberi. She was still depleted from walking the two miles to the staging area and staying awake for more than twenty-four hours. She stood in the back row, trying to conceal that she felt off balance.

Dorothy abruptly fainted. She regained consciousness as the nurses helped her up. They brushed the sandy dirt from her uniform and eased her into a chair a soldier had rushed over. The admiral paused until he regained the women's attention. Then he continued to deliver his remarks while the camera bulbs burst. Dorothy hunched over and laboriously breathed through an open mouth. Eldene inched toward her ailing friend, careful to keep her eyes on the admiral. The Seventh Fleet, he told them proudly, was "MacArthur's Navy."

Admiral Kinkaid invited the women to a special luncheon held in their honor. In the meantime, they were welcome to visit the paymaster. During their internment, the navy had changed its policy so that nurses were considered commissioned officers. Dorothy and the others were given the rank of ensign, with the exception of Laura Cobb, who was recognized as a lieutenant commander. The navy was also compensating the women for their years of service as prisoners of war. The women expressed relief as they waited to see the paymaster.

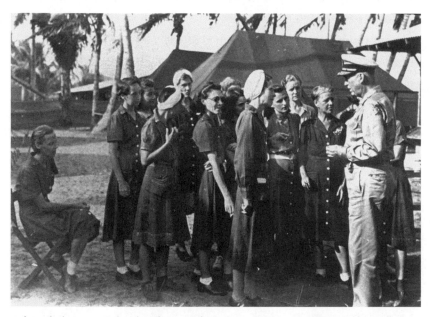

Admiral Thomas Kinkaid welcomes the navy nurses to Leyte. Dorothy Still is seated because she passed out during the greeting. *Courtesy of Bureau of Medicine and Surgery*

They had served as nurses for more than three years without guarantee the navy would pay them for their efforts. The back wages were both recognition for their work and hope for the future. Mary Rose later commented how she and her fiancé had left Los Baños holding a few cans of corned beef and little else. But they soon had cash. Mary Rose received back pay of about $6,400,* and her fiancé, a US Treasury worker, was paid a per diem for his years of imprisonment. The couple owned nothing, but the influx of cash gave them a quick start at building a new life.

Dorothy remained in her chair as the paymaster tried to sort through the women's owed wages. She was approached by a lieutenant she'd known at Cavite, a man she dated just once. She had not felt a strong connection at the time and had declined further invitations. Almost four years later, the lieutenant still burned from the rejection. He knew Dorothy had been a POW, yet his wounded pride overrode his sympathy. He wanted Dorothy to know he had married a beautiful Filipina woman and was so happy. Dorothy chose not to respond. She sensed that he wanted her to regret not pursuing him when she had the chance. Goldia interrupted the lieutenant's bragging. The women were due at the luncheon with the admiral.

Dorothy took a fabric square and folded it into a triangle. She wrapped the scarf around her head, tucking the ends into small openings at the top. She resembled the model in the famous "We Can Do It" posters the war department had released three years prior. She'd missed that cultural icon, as well as so many other events that defined American life in the 1940s. As she filed into the mess hall for lunch with the

---

* About $90,000 today. Mary Rose also noted that the nurses were not given the rent or subsistence payments the navy gave men. If they had, the navy nurses would have received an additional $2,600, about $37,000 more in today's currency.

admiral, she realized the nurses had little in common with their dining companions. The men were high-ranking naval officers, well-fed
men in their fifties.

The women were encouraged to mix among the naval officers.
Dorothy used the opportunity to distance herself from her chief nurse.
She was still not fond of Cobb and she was tired of being under
the woman's command. Dorothy lit a cigarette and looked around
the narrow room. The conversation was awkward until Peg joked
about attending a function with high-level officers wearing a ratty
denim uniform. The women had once worn uniforms made from
dungarees, she said—could the officers believe it? The humor seemed
to lighten the mood and helped the conversation build. In moments of
silence, the nurses plied the men with questions about current events
at home. Who was the vice president? Who won the World Series?
What was the biggest film last year?

Dorothy chewed her filet mignon, feeling uneasy as her stomach
lurched from the density of the meat. She wasn't ready for steak, she
sadly realized. She took slow, careful bites of her mashed potatoes
and peas.

A few seats down, nurse Mary Rose noticed Dorothy wasn't touch-
ing her steak. "What's the matter, Dottie?" Mary Rose asked. "Aren't
you going to finish your steak?"

Dorothy shook her head. "It's too rich."

"Pass it over," Mary Rose instructed. She cut into the extra piece
of meat and finished it off.

Other nurses were also doubling up on their food intake. Earlier
in the morning, a soldier had invited Peg and Bertha to the commis-
sary and offered to treat them to a sweet. The women had apple pie
and ice cream. Cobb didn't mind her nurses eating extra. She wanted
them to gain weight in a slow and healthy manner. But she tried to
block the navy's attempt to serve her nurses alcohol. "My girls haven't
had any liquor!" Cobb scolded.

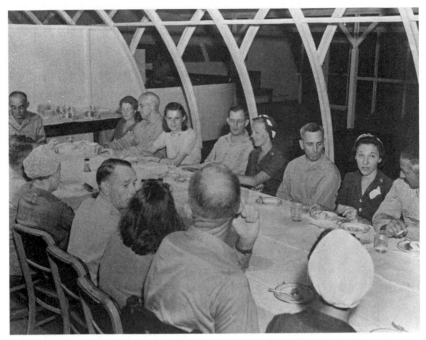

The navy nurses having lunch with officers at Leyte. *Seated at the far side of the table, left to right:* Mary Rose Harrington, Mary Chapman, Dorothy Still (wearing head scarf), Helen Gorzelanski. *Courtesy of Bureau of Medicine and Surgery*

Bertha had to stop herself from reacting. She was forty years old and she wasn't a *girl*. And as a freshly released prisoner of war, she would have a cocktail if she wanted to. She didn't happen to want a drink at the moment, but she wanted the option. Mary Rose risked irritating her superior and had a beer.

Nurse Basilia seemed to care for none of it. Jerry had not been invited to the luncheon and she was required to spend an hour among naval officers when she'd rather be with her husband. Basilia was likely pleased it was all over when the meal ended and Admiral Kinkaid wished the women well. They were due on a cargo plane to Guam. The admiral apologized in advance that the plane would be very cold.

The army nurses had winter uniforms the navy nurses could borrow. Although none of the women wanted to wear the other corps' uniform, no one chanced a declaration that she'd die before wearing those. It had taken far too long to get rid of those damned dungarees.

The nurses loaded themselves onto the cargo plane with several navy officers who also required transport to Guam. The officers watched the women with fascination. As soon as the plane gained altitude, the women pulled out the ration boxes they'd been given and worked their way through each item. They took small bites, eating slowly and steadily. The officers remarked that it was like flying with a bunch of rabbits.

The next few days brought a series of plane rides and media appearances. After Guam, the women flew to the Marshall Islands, then the Johnston Islands, and finally Pearl Harbor. The nurses were expected to grant gracious interviews in which they complained not one bit about the US Navy but tore into the enemy. Lieutenant Commander Cobb gave a few reporters what they wanted when she told them what she planned to do after her ninety-day leave. "I want to return to the Philippines," Cobb told a correspondent. "If I don't, I'll be all finished with this war. I've been on the receiving end too long. Now I'd like to be on the other side."

Peg offered a similar narrative. "We want to dish it out a while."

At Pearl Harbor, the nurses were asked to pose for a series of photographs in which they feigned delight in rediscovering everyday comforts. The purpose of the photos seemed to be to assure American newspaper readers that the women were being fixed—as if chocolate, cosmetics, and hair conditioner were all they needed to right themselves. Helen was the gamest of the group, though she might have been mocking the photographers more than they realized. She posed with Dorothy in front of a vanity, as if to demonstrate that a return to beauty standards was soothing to their psyche. She pushed her fingertips into a mattress top to model her joy at sleeping on a box spring. And she reclined on a twin bed with Eldene and paged through a magazine.

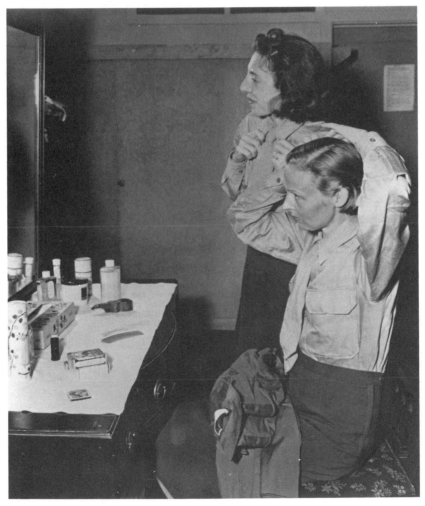

Helen Gorzelanski *(standing)* and Dorothy Still pose in front of a vanity for photographers. *Courtesy of Bureau of Medicine and Surgery*

In truth, the women were irritated by the attention and eager to go home. Bertha had to stop herself from snapping at a reporter in Pearl Harbor who rushed onto the tarmac to ask questions. They were given leis and required to stand next to the plane and smile, as if all was well. But all was *not* well. Each woman had a raging case of post-traumatic stress disorder. They didn't need chocolate creams or the latest copy of *Cosmopolitan* magazine. They needed trauma counseling and group therapy sessions.

The navy physicians were only trained to diagnose the nurses' physical ailments. At Oak Knoll Naval Hospital in Oakland, California, the women underwent medical examinations and received treatment plans. Then they were due at a reception with naval officers. It seemed they were public property and there was only one way to frame their suffering: as a mild hardship stoically endured. The newspaper coverage downplayed their suffering, often describing the nurses as medical witnesses to the other prisoners' agony. Other reporters treated them like girls back from camp, describing them as "eager for cosmetics" and willing to eat anything, including Spam. Readers were apparently meant to chuckle at such a comment.

But the nurses did have their own agony, and it was exasperated by their hasty separation from one another. As much as the other women often grated on Dorothy's nerves, they were the only ones who truly understood what she had endured. After Oakland, the women were sent to their respective homes for their ninety-day leaves, and then on to other assignments. Dorothy, Eldene, Edwina, and Mary Rose went to Southern California. In the Midwest, Mary Francis went to Chicago, Susie to Iowa, and Goldia to Minnesota. In the Great Plains, Cobb returned to Kansas and Helen to Nebraska. Bertha went up to Oregon. Basilia moved to Texas with Jerry. And Peg was sent to an East Coast hospital for extended care. She had tuberculosis and the prognosis was grim. Peg was told she should not expect to live for more than five years.

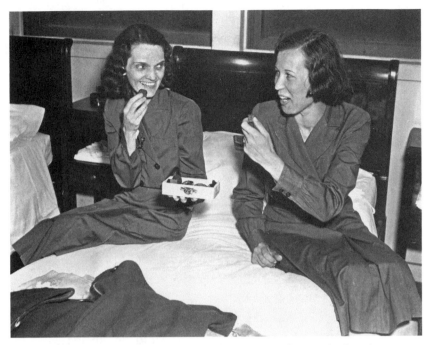

Peg Nash *(left)* and Bertha Evans pose for photographers with chocolates.
Courtesy of Bureau of Medicine and Surgery

The navy permitted Peg to return home after she learned her mother was ill. The local newspaper printed her train's arrival time and a welcoming committee arranged to greet her. Almost five thousand people attended the parade. Peg went through the motions, meeting the mayor to receive keys to the city and stopping at her parish for a prayer service. After the town was finished celebrating her, Peg was finally able to visit her mother, whom she hadn't seen in more than five years. Why hadn't anyone thought *that* should be her first order of business?

The celebration of Peg's homecoming was exemplary of well-meaning people who lacked the social delicacy one should show a newly released prisoner of war. The women were constantly asked if they had been raped by the Japanese, and the people asking expected an honest answer, as if they were entitled to know. Other civilians shifted the conversation to themselves, telling the nurses about the deprivations they had experienced under war rationing. On several occasions during her leave, Dorothy had to listen to an oblivious civilian tell her about the difficulty of planning a weekly menu when ration cards limited meat and dairy purchases.

Callous comments made the nurses feel as though they weren't understood, and it made adjustment seem impossible. Dorothy felt depressed during the ninety-day leave and often burst into tears in moments she least expected it. The people who understood her best were the former inmates, but they were scattered across the country. Thomas, although he was only a bus ride away, might as well have been in another country. He was with his family, and her closest confidant was as good as dead.

Many former POWs struggled to adjust and felt alienated by having experienced something other people could not imagine. Naval surgeon Ferdinand Berley had been transferred from Bilibid to Japan on a "hell ship." After liberation, he began his journey home on a hospital vessel. The ship played movies in the evening, and Ferdinand wanted to join the activities and be part of the group. But his mind couldn't reconcile his years of torment with the placidity of sailors watching a film. Simply being away from the suffering wasn't enough. He cried when the room went dark. He moved into the corner and sobbed throughout the features. The other men distanced themselves. Ferdinand kept to himself.

Peg felt the same isolation. She was briefly confined to a tuberculosis sanitarium and then permitted to return home. She was haunted by her memories and felt as though her emotions were uncontrollable. Her stress increased in the autumn of 1945 when she learned that her fiancé had survived his ordeal in a Japanese prison camp. Peg reunited with Edwin Wood and tried to help him adjust to the shock of returning to the United States. But knowing her condition wasn't improving and she wasn't expected to live much longer, she canceled the wedding and urged Edwin to move on. He did so immediately. The following April, he was already engaged to another woman.

Peg later described herself as going crazy. The once-energetic woman was broken. It was an assessment the military was not interested in confirming. Mental anguish was reserved for men, although even for them diagnosis rarely led to treatment. The released prisoners suffered constant anxiety, which the navy described as "worrying over everything in reality." They had periods of depression and tormenting nightmares, and felt easily irritated. Some were exhausted by everyday life. Former inmates described themselves as having an inferiority complex or a lack of self-confidence. They were nervous in crowds, and they admitted that their own fatalistic comments made other people nervous.

Many did not expect to live a full life, and one anticipated he would be "an old man at forty." Former prisoners' hands shook. They woke up screaming in the night when the guards haunted their dreams. They snapped at their spouses, exploded at their children, and then hated themselves for the outbursts. They felt useless, as though they had contributed nothing to the war. Dorothy fought feelings of worthlessness. When the fog of self-doubt clouded her thoughts, she forgot that she had cared for thousands of prisoners when she herself was a patient.

The twelve anchors, the women who had kept others from drifting in the prison camps, were now feeling the weight of their efforts. Dorothy experienced momentary relief when she received the same orders as Eldene to report to Bethesda, Maryland. They drove across the country together in an old Hudson sedan. Their time in the car likely gave them an opportunity to remember their shared experience. But then Dorothy was plucked by the navy as a war bond speaker. She was sent to fundraising events throughout the East Coast and required to divulge her experiences to large audiences. Dorothy was agitated, and she continued to burst into tears unexpectedly. Wanting to be free from the attention, she put in a request to transfer to the naval base in Panama.

Dorothy found her own anchor in the turbulence. A friend from Southern California, Goldburn "Peck" Danner, was also a naval officer. He became her new confidant and she shared her difficulties. Peck urged Dorothy to see the navy psychiatrist. Peck believed the psychiatrist would grant Dorothy a medical discharge, which would place her on the retirement list. It was time, Peck urged, for Dorothy to leave the navy.

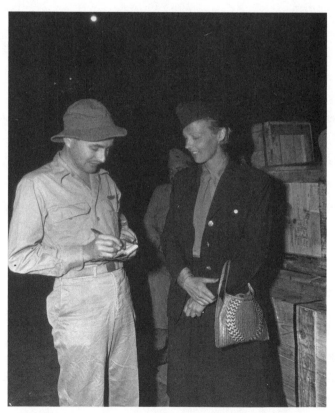

Dorothy Still grants an interview. *Courtesy of Bureau of Medicine and Surgery*

Dorothy followed through with the appointment. She sat in the physician's office, related her experience as a prisoner of war, and told him of some of the emotions she endured as a result. She told the doctor she'd been liberated on February 23, 1945.

"You lie," the doctor interrupted.

Dorothy stopped speaking. The doctor proceeded to tell Dorothy that February 23, 1945, was the famed date of the battle of Iwo Jima, when six US marines planted the flag at the top of Mount Suribachi. Those men, the doctor sneered, saw battle. They suffered. Dorothy was neither a soldier nor a sailor and she never went to battle. She was a fake!

Dorothy left the office shaking. She knew she was telling the truth, and she knew she had suffered through war. The bombing at Cavite. The taunting sentries at Santa Scholastica. The starvation at Santo Tomas and the murders at Los Baños. She was there. But she saw no point in pushing other people to understand a depth of despair that their limited minds could not handle. Dorothy resolved to protect herself from such unprovoked meanness. Her stories were now her own. She would keep them to herself.

Epilogue

———

I Hear You

IN JULY 1945, Henry Carpenter stared across the golf greens. The former Los Baños inmate was back in Manila trying to piece together his life. He lowered his golf club and fixated on a labor detail of Japanese POWs working nearby. The inmates were tasked with dismantling the ammunition depot the Japanese army had built on the golf course during the occupation. One of the inmates looked familiar to Henry. The stained teeth. The constant scowl. That man, Henry realized, was not some rank-and-file member of the Japanese Imperial Army. That man was responsible for his daily agony at Los Baños. It was Konishi.

Since fleeing from Los Baños and initiating his bloody campaign of revenge, Sadaaki Konishi had become a wanted war criminal. But he passed himself off as an ordinary member of the Japanese army when he was taken prisoner by Allied forces. He might have been repatriated to Japan if Henry hadn't spotted him on the golf course.

The US Army promptly pulled Konishi from the POW camp to face charges for crimes against humanity.

An investigator assigned to the army's war crimes department interviewed Konishi shortly after he was identified. Konishi denied deliberately starving the inmates. In the interview, the former supply officer claimed he was merely following orders when he restricted the rations. Konishi said he agreed that the amount fed to the Los Baños inmates was not enough to sustain a human being, but he asserted that he had protested to headquarters about the inadequate food supply. All of it, he claimed, was out of his control.

A man once so focused on commandeering the camp now acted as though he'd had no real authority. His lack of power, he maintained, was the reason he was unable to allow the inmates to leave the prison to forage for food. The investigator remained skeptical and forced Konishi to acknowledge that the Los Baños area was one of the most productive regions in the world for growing coconuts, bananas, and sweet potatoes. Konishi could have ordered his sentries to pluck nearby fruits or permitted the inmates to continue their gardens.

Konishi lied endlessly to his interrogator. He feigned ignorance, as though he was the last to know about anything that happened in the camp. He claimed he was only informed of Howard Hell's killing after the fact. And he swore he had nothing to do with the execution of George Louis.

The interrogator wasn't buying it. "Didn't you, as a matter of fact, hand your pistol to a guard who executed George Louis while you were standing there?" he demanded.

"Positively no," Konishi said to the interpreter. He continued to deny his wrongdoings, including the massacre of the Los Baños locals. His defense was he was only in the area to confiscate food.

At Konishi's trial, a five-member military commission voted secretly on six charges including starving inmates, slaughtering locals, and murdering George Louis. The commission found Konishi guilty on all counts and sentenced him to death. The execution was postponed several times, partly due to his lawyers claiming he had tuberculosis. Konishi was finally executed on April 30, 1949.

In the coming years, the war tribunals in both Europe and the South Pacific calculated the loss of life in enemy prisoner of war camps. Americans held in European camps by Nazis had a 1 percent mortality rate. Americans held in Japanese POW camps had about a 40 percent mortality rate. For the civilians imprisoned in Japanese camps, including the two dominated by Konishi, the death rate was 11 percent. The death rate of the Philippine forces was staggering. An estimated fifty-seven thousand Filipino soldiers died—almost half at Camp O'Donnell after the surrender of Bataan. As many as one million civilians, including the fifteen hundred Los Baños area residents, were killed during the war.

Konishi had tried his best to create a slow-motion death camp at both Santo Tomas and Los Baños. The navy nurses and their army counterparts resisted each day by providing medical services, even though they were in need of care themselves. All the navy, army, and civilian nurses survived the ordeal.

Navy nurse Ann Bernatitus arrived back in the United States in September 1942. She continued to provide nursing care during the war and served as chief nurse on a hospital ship, the USS *Relief*. After the war, Ann earned a specialization in occupational therapy. She remained in the navy until 1959 and retired with the rank of captain. After her retirement, Ann returned to her family's home in Wilkes-Barre, which had been built by her parents in 1905. She sold medical equipment and volunteered at a retirement home. She died in 2003 at the age of ninety-one.

After liberation, Dr. Dana Nance returned to the United States and was met on the boat dock by his wife, Anna. Dana promptly wrote the US Navy and urged officials to honor the navy nurses with a unit commendation. Although his efforts failed, the navy did reward the women with a Bronze Star for meritorious achievement in a combat zone as well as the Prisoner of War Medal. The women also received several army honors. Dana established a private practice in Tennessee and later retired to Mexico. He died in 1987 at the age of eighty-three.

Dorothy's army nurse friend, Gwendolyn Henshaw, returned to California after the war and promptly married a prisoner from Santo Tomas. Her husband, James F. Perrine, was an oil company executive and the two moved to Hong Kong. In 1960, James suffered a cardiac incident and died in the ambulance at the age of fifty-eight. The cause of death was listed as heart disease, a condition that congressional researchers found was common among the survivors of Japanese POW camps. Gwendolyn returned to California and remarried in 1963. She and her second husband were married for thirty-six years, until both died in 1999 just a few months apart.

Gwendolyn's husband was not the only one whose medical condition was aggravated by the prison camps. Basilia Torres Steward's husband, Jerry, also suffered from his war wounds as well as a heart condition. The navy retired him in November 1946 with the rank of rear admiral. Although grateful for the honor of his high rank, Jerry felt depressed by the idea of retirement. He decided to run for the Texas legislature. He was elected and served from 1948 to 1951. As a politician's wife, Basilia was highly regarded in the newspapers for her service during the war. Jerry died in 1960 and Basilia remained in Texas until her death in 1994 at age eighty. She was honored with a Bronze Star from the navy as well as the WWII Victory Medal. Although the Bronze Star was "technically" only for members of the navy nurse corps, the US secretary of the navy wisely ignored such a detail. Basilia also received the Philippine Defense and Liberation Medals from the Philippine government.

Of the navy nurses, Susie Pitcher had been one of the most ill during internment. After liberation, she remained in the navy and was stationed at the Great Lakes Naval Base in northern Illinois. She died from leukemia in 1951 at the age of fifty. She was the first of the twelve anchors to die, and the one who died the youngest.

Nebraskan Helen Gorzelanski's life was also cut short. She left the navy after the war, got married, and lived with her husband in California, near Napa. In 1972, Helen and her husband, Arthur Hunter, were driving on a highway on a Sunday afternoon. A twenty-three-year-old drunk driver crashed her pickup truck into Helen's vehicle. A witness described the drunk driver as speeding at eighty-five miles per hour and swerving across lanes. Helen was sixty-four.

Chief Nurse Laura Cobb had hidden her ailments in the camps. She suffered from painful arthritis as well as a heart condition. In 1947, no longer able to bear the pain, she retired from the navy with the rank of lieutenant commander. She served as a nurse in a civilian hospital for the next two decades. Cobb enjoyed fifteen years of retirement in California before her death in 1981 at the age of eighty-nine.

Peg Nash continued to suffer from tuberculosis, and the navy gave her a medical release in 1946. She moved to Southern California on a physician's advice and began working at a children's hospital. She later worked in student health at the University of Southern California. She was friendly with the students and willing to tell interested listeners about her experiences in the war. Though she hadn't been expected to live for more than five years after the war, Peg worked until she was old enough to retire, then volunteered as a home nurse for elderly patients. She died in 1994 at the age of eighty-one.

Like Peg, dietitian Bertha Evans did not marry her fiancé from Cavite. She remained in the navy, advanced to the rank of commander, and served as the chief nurse at the naval hospital in Bremerton. She also served in the Korean War. She later married a man named Egean St. Pierre and left the navy. She died in 2001 at the age of ninety-six. Of the twelve nurses, she lived to the oldest age.

Edwina Todd also had a successful career in the navy. She served for thirty years and rose to the rank of captain, the highest of any of the anchors. During the Korean War, she served as chief nurse on the USS *Consolation*. She went on to earn a bachelor's in nursing education as well as a master's in nursing service administration. She retired from the navy in 1966 and was active with civic organizations until her death in 1996.

Mary Chapman returned to Chicago and was greeted on the tarmac by her parents and younger siblings. She promptly married her fiancé, William R. Hays, who had been wounded and sent home early in the war. She died at the age of fifty-five in 1969 after becoming ill the year before.

Goldia O'Haver also had a wedding shortly after her liberation. Goldia married Robert Heath Merrill, the army mechanic she'd met at Los Baños, after he arrived in California in May 1945. She retired from the navy the following year and the couple moved to Apple Valley, California. She died in 1977 at the age of seventy-four.

Mary Rose Harrington married a Los Baños inmate as well. She wed Page Nelson on April 13, 1945. The couple was aware their wedding date was Friday the Thirteenth, but they were eager to marry after years of being denied. Page continued his career with the US Treasury. Mary Rose became a mother of four children. She remained active with nursing as a Red Cross volunteer. For forty years she volunteered with bloodmobiles and administered polio vaccinations. She also testified to Congress pertaining women in the military. She died in 1999 at age eighty-five.

Eldene Paige found peace after the war. She returned to her family farm near Paradise, California, and lived with her mother. Her nieces and nephews remembered her as a kind woman who was fun to be around. They followed her around the farm, helping her to feed chickens and do light chores. The only time they were not allowed to trail her was when she hosted the Los Baños nurses every summer. About five women came each year, and they wanted to be alone, perhaps to discuss their memories. Eldene died in 2004 at the age of ninety. She was the last of the twelve anchors to die.

In 1946, Dorothy was stationed in Panama when she accepted a marriage proposal from her friend and confidant Peck Danner. That June, she purchased a car and had it shipped to New Orleans. Peck met Dorothy in New Orleans and the couple drove the new car to California, eloping along the way. They moved to a quiet patch of land in Glendale, where Peck tried egg farming. Their first child, a daughter, was born in 1947. A son followed two years later.

Dorothy focused on her young family, but Thomas Terrill proved to be a disruption. He tried to maintain a distant friendship and even invited himself and his family to the Danners' ranch. The visit brought back too many memories, and Dorothy retreated to the back of the house to cry. Peck gently encouraged Dorothy to sever the friendship so that she could move on.

In time, Dorothy found she was moving on. Peck returned to his previous career in sound engineering and took a job with CBS. The family moved to a three-bedroom home in Glendale, and Dorothy became pregnant with their third child, a son. Peck, Dorothy found, was a remarkable and gentle man. He was the strength Dorothy needed.

In August 1956, Peck traveled to San Francisco for CBS to cover the Republican National Convention and the renomination of President Dwight D. Eisenhower. While there, Peck suffered a coronary hemorrhage and died at the age of forty-eight. Back in Glendale,

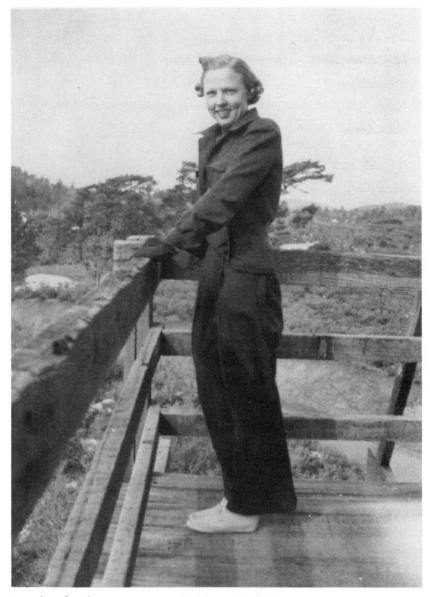

Dorothy after the war. *Courtesy of Bureau of Medicine and Surgery*

Dorothy learned her beloved husband was gone. She was a widow at the age of forty-one with a nine-year-old daughter, a seven-year-old son, and another son due in two months.

Dorothy, ever the survivor, continued on. She moved her young family to Carlsbad, California, and bought a house one block from the ocean. The beach became her children's playground. She returned to nursing while also managing the family home. Her children recall her as loving and supportive. She was also remarkably resilient. When the house needed a patio, she leveled the area, poured the sand foundation, and laid the bricks by herself.

In the late 1960s, mutual friends realized they knew both Thomas and Dorothy. Thomas was also single by this time, and friends encouraged the two to communicate. Dorothy was initially cautious, but she sent a short note. Thomas responded by sending a tape cassette with a recorded message. He asked Dorothy to send back a recording so he might hear her voice again. One afternoon, Dorothy's older son came for a visit and paused to watch his mother through the kitchen window. Dorothy was intently listening to the tape recorder and quickly hit the stop button when her son appeared. After a bit of pressing, Dorothy admitted she had a friend from the war with whom she might reconnect.

Thomas and Dorothy indeed found their way back to each other, and the couple married in a ceremony in his sister's hospital room. His sister was not well and wanted to see Thomas and Dorothy wed before she passed. Thomas and Dorothy enjoyed more than fifteen years together before he died in 1986.

In the 1990s, Dorothy began thinking more about her experiences in the war. Decades earlier, *Life* magazine had published the photograph of her and Eldene nursing on top of the amtrac. As a child, Dorothy's daughter found the magazine and asked her mother about the war, but Dorothy hesitated to discuss her experiences. The 1990s, however, brought a collective interest in preserving veterans' experiences. Authors, historians, and documentary makers were interested in recording personal histories before the Greatest Generation left this world.

In 1991, Dorothy gave an extensive, twenty-six-hundred-word oral history to the Bureau of Medicine and Surgery. She also participated in a documentary about the military nurse POWs. After years of being silenced, she wanted to tell people what she had experienced. Several of the other nurses, including Mary Rose, Peg, and Bertha, also gave oral histories. Peg mentioned she was disappointed the bombing at Cavite was rarely mentioned in history. The victims had endured a savage death, and Peg wished their plight was better understood. The women suffered as well, but there was little space to tell the story.

In 1995, Dorothy sought to change that. She wrote a memoir, *What a Way to Spend a War*. She initially wrote it in the third-person, calling herself Millie. She was haunted by the psychiatrist who told her she'd never suffered and shouldn't complain. She also didn't see herself as a hero and didn't want to suggest to readers that she had done something remarkable. The historian at the Naval Institute worked with Dorothy to make her memoir a historical document. Although she made changes to her manuscript at the historian's suggestion, she resisted revealing for readers what she had endured as a POW. In her writing, she often described how she felt but hesitated to put it in a larger context. She clearly wanted to tell her story, yet it seemed she wasn't convinced she had the right to be heard.

Dorothy died in 2001 at the age of eighty-six. She was buried with full honors at Arlington National Cemetery. As a retired lieutenant commander, she was entitled to six white horses pulling her casket atop a limber and caisson. The three-volley salute was followed by the playing of taps. The American flag was folded and presented to her adult children.

Following the burial, the Navy Nurse Corps had something planned: they had arranged for the Passing of the Flag. This ceremony is reserved for flag officers only—rear admirals or higher. Dorothy's rank of lieutenant commander was three levels below the cutoff, so

Dorothy was technically not eligible, but the corps realized that she indeed was worthy. Dorothy Still, navy nurse and POW, nursed to the end of her captivity. And her successors in the nurse corps passed the flag in her honor. And in doing so they said, *I hear you*.

Acknowledgments

I FOUND DOROTHY'S MEMOIR on a top shelf at my local library. One of my most pleasurable pastimes is to wander library aisles and greedily pick off titles that pique my interest. I immediately felt a connection with Dorothy. I wanted her story to be fully told the way she likely intended but hesitated because that damn psychiatrist still haunted her doubts.

Researching and writing this book took almost two years, not including the editing process. As a journalist, I prefer to deal with primary sources and I have a list of people to thank for helping me to research this story and give these heroic women their due. First, I express gratitude to Dorothy's children—Dan, Margie, and Martin. Thank you so kindly for answering my many questions and making this book possible.

André Sobocinski, navy historian with the Bureau of Medicine and Surgery, provided me with an endless amount of oral history transcripts, medical expertise, photographs, records, and general guidance. One of the trickiest aspects of this book was keeping the medical knowledge limited to December 1941. Mr. Sobocinski was an amazing resource in helping me stay within these confines. No question was too small for him and I am grateful for his expertise, professionalism, and patience. I should also note that Mr. Sobocinski was the historian who recorded Dorothy's oral history in 1991. Thank you, Mr. Sobocinski, for giving this wonderful nurse a forum in which she felt welcome to fully express herself.

My quest for primary sources drew heavily on my local library. The Oak Park Public Library is a profound community resource. At times I needed a particular book or memoir from the 1940s that was not available locally, and the interlibrary loan service always came through for me. Most specifically, thank you to the one librarian who finagled me out of that unfortunate situation regarding Juanita Redmond's 1943 memoir—I accidentally kept the book three months past the due date. I was pretty sure I'd have to call the other library with my checking account's routing number, but my Oak Park librarian smoothed it over for me.

Also thank you to the University of Illinois-Chicago for having an open and wonderful system that allowed me to access many medical journals from the 1930s and 1940s. UIC has an amazing system in which you can chat with an online librarian to make sure the text is available before you make the trip. I also appreciate Bjorn Paige and his family for answering my questions.

This project would not have been possible without Lisa Reardon. She changed my life in 2015 when she agreed to take on my book about Sabella Nitti. She also saw the value in Dorothy's story, even when it was just a beginning idea that I brought up in a phone call. Lisa championed this project and made it possible to tell the story of Dorothy and the twelve anchors, who have often been confused with the Angels of Bataan or completely forgotten.

I also thank the team at Chicago Review Press. Publisher Cynthia Sherry has been an advocate for my work and has created an amazing space where women's stories matter. Thank you to my editor

Jerome Pohlen for taking me on and adding me to your impressive list. Thank you to my production editor, Devon Freeny, for polishing and improving my work. And thank you to my patient publicity manager, Olivia Aguilar. I'm sure my color-coded spreadsheets with ideas were exhausting.

On a personal note, I have so many people to thank. I have a list of friends who supported me in every way—I look forward to thanking you in person. Thank you to my friends and family who listened to my endless rehashing of my research. I had some difficulty processing much of what I read. For months, I had terrible dreams about prison guards lighting inmates on fire. I also felt stunned by many of the oral histories I read. In particular, I struggled with the prisoners' accounts of trying to normalize their lives. The Palawan massacre survivor, Rufus W. Smith, spoke of getting hold of a baseball and considering a game. He struck me as so young and vulnerable. Similarly, Dr. Ferdinand Berley's account of crying on the ship ride home put me into empathy overload and I admit I recounted these stories during social events. So . . . um . . . sorry about that.

On a much lighter note, I give special gratitude to Mia the Chihuahua and Daisy the Rescue Wonder for their expert companionship. Daisy is a very good sport and she let me hold her paw after bad dreams. Mia is not to be disturbed during the overnight hours. But she's a grade-A listener with a great doggy head tilt.

I thank the Le Beau and Lucchesi families for all their support.

Much love to my mother- and father-in-law, Rosa and Michael.

Special gratitude to Suzie and Tana. I look forward to our weekly visits. I learn so much from your wisdom, Tana.

Additional acknowledgment to Adina, Marda, Michelle, Glen, and Joe. Your love and support are incredible. I believe that one day I will look back on this time in my life and think these were my best years because I had all of you.

All my love to my parents, Joel and Francine, who have given me a lifetime of love and support. I am at a loss for words, because there is too much to say. I'll have to let Elton John say it for me: "I hope you don't mind that I put down in words how wonderful life is while you're in the world."

I dedicated this book to my grandfather Leon J. Le Beau, PhD. He was born in 1919 in a French Canadian community in Illinois and did not speak English until his parents moved to the Chicago area. He was a child of the Depression who picked up fallen coal along the railroad tracks to burn in his family's furnace. One year, he sold magazine subscriptions and earned points to purchase the only Christmas gifts his siblings received. (He selected a laboratory kit for himself.) In December 1941, he was a junior at Elmhurst College preparing to transfer to the University of Illinois' dental program. He joined the army after the attack on Pearl Harbor. He was with the Fifth Army's Medical Laboratory, and also served as a medic. He was part of the first wave into Japan after the surrender. After the war, he received his PhD in microbiology at the University of Illinois, where he served as a professor. He was a fast-moving optimist who always looked forward. We miss him.

And as always, I dedicate this book to my husband, Michael. I love you so much. I can't put it all into words, so I shall have Wild Cub do it for me: "I hear it call in the center of it all. . . . You're the love of my life, the love of my life."

Notes

1. I'd Die Before I Wore Those

Dorothy's room: Danner, *What a Way to Spend a War*; description taken from photographs from the Bureau of Medicine and Surgery.

Bertha hears of attack: Bureau of Medicine and Surgery, "Recollections of Ann Bernatitus"; Bureau of Medicine and Surgery, "Interview with Bertha Evans."

Army sends up planes: Carter and Mueller, *Combat Chronology*.

Bertha reports attack: Bureau of Medicine and Surgery, "Interview with Bertha Evans"; Bureau of Medicine and Surgery, "Recollections of Ann Bernatitus."

"Dottie! Wake up!" through *ordered her nurses into uniform*: Danner, *What a Way to Spend a War*; Bureau of Medicine and Surgery, "Oral History with Dorothy Still Danner."

Dorothy preparing in her room: Danner, *What a Way to Spend a War*; photographs of navy nurse uniforms supplied by Bureau of Medicine and Surgery, nos. 09-8156-1, 09-8164, BuAer 178052, and BuAer 178350.

traded mixed expressions through *"You girls ready for war?"*: Danner, *What a Way to Spend a War*; US Census 1930, Lake County, IL, roll 529, p. 29A, enumeration district 0064, FHL microfilm 2340264.

Bertha's boat anecdote and physical description: Bureau of Medicine and Surgery, "Interview with Bertha Evans"; photograph from Bureau of Medicine and Surgery, no. 09-8156-11.

Reporting for duty and running to the hospital: Danner, *What a Way to Spend a War*.

Dorothy's mother pushes nursing school and Great Depression unemployment: Danner, *What a Way to Spend a War*; Bureau of Medicine and Surgery, "Oral History with Dorothy Still Danner"; Bureau of Labor Statistics, "Series D 85-86, Unemployment: 1890 to 1970," in *Historical Statistics of the United States, Colonial Times to 1970*, pt. 1 (Washington, DC: US Government Printing Office, 1975), 135.

an exclusive honorary: Burbank High School, *The Ceralus* 21 (1931).

Nursing school and graduation, low wages, and contract struggles: Danner, *What a Way to Spend a War*; Bureau of Medicine and Surgery, "Interview with Margaret Nash."

Applying to the navy: Danner, *What a Way to Spend a War*; "The Federal Government Nursing Services," *American Journal of Nursing* 37, no. 11 (1937): 335–341.

It seemed that every newspaper: Author analysis of front-page headlines from December 13, 1937, through January 15, 1938.

Rape of Nanking and US reaction: Iris Chang, *The Rape of Nanking: The Forgotten Holocaust of World War II* (New York: Basic Books, 1997).

US preparedness: *Reports of the Secretary of War to the President* (Washington, DC: US Government Printing Office, 1938); *Reports of the Secretary of War to the President* (Washington, DC: US Government Printing Office, 1939).

transferred from San Diego through *very good assignment*: Danner, *What a Way to Spend a War*; Bureau of Medicine and Surgery, "Oral History with Dorothy Still Danner."

eleven-year timeline: Franklin D. Roosevelt: "Proclamation 2148: Establishment of the Commonwealth of the Philippines," November 14, 1935, available at American Presidency Project, www.presidency.ucsb.edu /node/208272.

Dorothy's good-bye to her family: Danner, *What a Way to Spend a War*.

"Pearl Harbor has been bombed": Bureau of Medicine and Surgery, "Interview with Margaret Nash."

mixed reactions through *tethered in place*: Danner, *What a Way to Spend a War*; Bureau of Medicine and Surgery, "Oral History with Ferdinand Berley"; Redmond, *I Served on Baatan*.

Japan had signed: Convention Relative to the Treatment of Prisoners of War, Geneva, July 27, 1929; Convention on the Opening of Hostilities, The Hague, October 18, 1907.

Evacuation of hospital: Danner, *What a Way to Spend a War*; Kentner, "Daily Journal of Events."

Dorothy and iron lung patients: Bureau of Medicine and Surgery, "Interview with Mary Rose Harrington."

A jittery current: Danner, *What a Way to Spend a War*.

Japan attacks: Carter and Mueller, *Combat Chronology*; Douglas MacArthur, *Reports of General MacArthur: Japanese Operations in the Southwest Pacific Area*, vol. 2, pt. 1 (Washington, DC: Department of the Army, 1966); Col. Ruby G. Bradley, "Prisoners in the Far East," Army Nurse Corps Historical Documentation, 2010, Office of Medical History, US Army Medical Department.

Peg Nash background: Bureau of Medicine and Surgery, "Interview with Margaret Nash"; World War II Veterans Compensation Applications, Records of the Department of Military and Veterans Affairs, RG 19, series 19.92.

Food at Cavite and air raid begins: Danner, *What a Way to Spend a War*; Bureau of Medicine and Surgery, "Oral History with Ferdinand Berley."

Nurses ordered to shelter: Danner, *What a Way to Spend a War*.

Attack on Clark Field: Carter and Mueller, *Combat Chronology*; MacArthur, *Reports of General MacArthur*; Edmonds, *They Fought with What They Had*.

Two nurses were being transferred through *pulling on the dungarees*: Danner, *What a Way to Spend a War*; Bureau of Medicine and Surgery, "Recollections of Ann Bernatitus"; Bureau of Medicine and Surgery, "Interview with Margaret Nash."

Ward preparations: Danner, *What a Way to Spend a War*; US Navy, *Handbook of the Hospital Corps* (Washington, DC: Bureau of Medicine and Surgery, 1939); Kentner, "Daily Journal of Events"; Bureau of Medicine and Surgery, "Interview with Margaret Nash"; Todd, "Nursing Under Fire."

Dorothy in the ward: Danner, *What a Way to Spend a War*.

Pearl Harbor destruction: "U.S. Census Bureau History: Pearl Harbor," US Census Bureau official website, December 2016, www.census.gov /history/www/homepage_archive/2016/december_2016.html.

Pearl Harbor casualties: Schwartz, "Experiences in Battle"; Claude S. Beck and John H. Powers, "Burns Treated by Tannic Acid," *Annals of Surgery* 84, no. 1 (1926): 19–36; medical officer in command of Naval Hospital, Pearl Harbor, letter to chief of Bureau of Navigation, December 22, 1941; medical officer in command of Naval Hospital, Pearl Harbor, letter to chief of Bureau of Medicine and Surgery, January 16, 1942.

2. Oh My God, This Is Really War

Overnight air raids drills: Danner, *What a Way to Spend a War*; Kentner, "Daily Journal of Events."

Morning shift: Danner, *What a Way to Spend a War*.

State of navy fleet: Gordon, *Fighting for MacArthur*.

braced for the attack: Danner, *What a Way to Spend a War*; Bureau of Medicine and Surgery, "Interview with Bertha Evans."

Bombing of yard: Gordon, *Fighting for MacArthur*; Danner, *What a Way to Spend a War*; Cressman, *Official Chronology*.

Eldene Paige: Danner, *What a Way to Spend a War*; Death Record 570-12-1044, Death Master List, US Social Security Administration; "State Summary of War Casualties from World War II for Navy, Marine Corps, and Coast Guard Personnel," Records of the Bureau of Naval Personnel, RG 24, roll ww2c_27, National Archives, College Park, MD.

"No point in waiting any longer" through *downed trees*: Danner, *What a Way to Spend a War*; digital archives from Roy Gerald King Papers, Institute on World War II and the Human Experience, Florida State University,

Tallahassee, FL; US Army Signal Corps, "Attack on Manila Harbor" (film), *Combat Bulletin* 40 (1945).

Cavite, she realized through *"Oh my God, this is really war"*: Danner, *What a Way to Spend a War*; Bureau of Medicine and Surgery, "Oral History with Dorothy Still Danner"; Bureau of Medicine and Surgery, "Interview with Margaret Nash."

Description of injuries: Danner, *What a Way to Spend a War*; Todd, "Nursing Under Fire"; Bureau of Medicine and Surgery, "Interview with Bertha Evans"; Bureau of Medicine and Surgery, "Interview with Margaret Nash."

Burn victim treatment: Josephine Bennett, "The Nursing Care of Burned Patients," *American Journal of Nursing* 37, no. 12 (1937): 1334.

Description of burns: Danner, *What a Way to Spend a War*; Bureau of Medicine and Surgery, "Interview with Margaret Nash"; Bertha Harmer, *The Principles and Practice of Nursing* (New York: Macmillan, 1930).

Administering morphine: Author's electronic correspondence with André B. Sobocinski, US Navy Bureau of Medicine and Surgery, September 28, 2017; US Navy, *Handbook of the Hospital Corps*.

She inspected patients through *taken to the morgue*: Danner, *What a Way to Spend a War*.

much deeper than it appeared: Todd, "Nursing Under Fire."

Civilian arrivals, Dorothy taking charge: Danner, *What a Way to Spend a War*; Bureau of Medicine and Surgery, "Interview with Bertha Evans"; Bureau of Medicine and Surgery, "Interview with Margaret Nash"; Todd, "Nursing Under Fire"; Kentner, "Daily Journal of Events."

A little boy asked through *those who were already dead*: Danner, *What a Way to Spend a War*; Bureau of Medicine and Surgery, "Oral History with Dorothy Still Danner"; Bureau of Medicine and Surgery, "Interview with Margaret Nash."

3. Everything Under Control

Lipstick on foreheads: Bureau of Medicine and Surgery, "Interview with Mary Rose Harrington."

"Line them up" through *a growing heap*: Bureau of Medicine and Surgery, "Interview with Margaret Nash"; Bureau of Medicine and Surgery, "Oral History with Ferdinand Berley."

Nursing assignments: Bureau of Medicine and Surgery, "Interview with Mary Rose Harrington."

Surgical team: Bureau of Medicine and Surgery, "Oral History with Ferdinand Berley."

Unconscious patient revives: Bureau of Medicine and Surgery, "Interview with Bertha Evans"; Bureau of Medicine and Surgery, "Interview with Margaret Nash"; Lt. Comm. Arthur M. McMaster, "Treatment of Cardiovascular Emergencies," *US Naval Medicine Bulletin* 39, no. 1 (1941): 74.

the navy stopped paychecks: Glusman, *Conduct Under Fire.*

a terrifying warning: Todd, "Nursing Under Fire."

one called for her softly through *could see her red eyes*: Danner, *What a Way to Spend a War*; Bureau of Medicine and Surgery, "Oral History with Dorothy Still Danner."

Dorothy stood on the dock through *fully comprehend the loss*: Danner, *What a Way to Spend a War.*

Patrol torpedo boat: Danner, *What a Way to Spend a War*; *Jane's Fighting Ships of World War II* (London: Random House, 1989).

Combining of staff, assignment to Jai Alai Building: Kentner, "Daily Journal of Events."

Transformation of Jai Alai Building: Danner, *What a Way to Spend a War.*

Newspaper response to Cavite bombing: Author analysis of headlines from December 11, 1941.

Navy nurses sending telegrams: Danner, *What a Way to Spend a War.*

Dorothy's telegram: Dorothy Still, telegram to William Still, December 13, 1941, courtesy of Bureau of Medicine and Surgery.

Dorothy's ride home: Danner, *What a Way to Spend a War.*

MacArthur had holed up: Sides, *Ghost Soldiers.*

Washington conference: US Department of State, *Foreign Relations of the United States: Conferences at Washington, 1941–1942, and Casablanca, 1943* (Washington, DC: US Government Printing Office, 1958), 251; Matloff and Snell, *US Army in World War II.*

"Europe First" plan: Matloff and Snell, *US Army in World War II*; MacArthur, *Reminiscences*.

War Plan Orange, its failures, and the navy's departure: Morton, *War in the Pacific*; Casey, *Engineers in Theatre Operations*; Hart, *War in the Pacific*.

At the Jai Alai through *their own death sentences*: Danner, *What a Way to Spend a War*; Bureau of Medicine and Surgery, "Oral History with Dorothy Still Danner."

4. Banzai

Aftermath of navy departure: Danner, *What a Way to Spend a War*; Kentner, "Daily Journal of Events."

Ann Bernatitus's departure: Bureau of Medicine and Surgery, "Recollections of Ann Bernatitus"; Kentner, "Daily Journal of Events"; Danner, *What a Way to Spend a War*.

Burning of flag: Todd, "Nursing Under Fire."

Bicycle troops: Bureau of Medicine and Surgery, "Oral History with Pharmacist's Mate Donald Tapscott."

Release of prisoners: Danner, *What a Way to Spend a War*.

Staff numbers: Kentner, "Daily Journal of Events."

Background of Basilia Torres Steward: "Petitions for Naturalization, 1906–1981," Records of District Courts of the United States, 1685–2009, RG 21, petition no. 2353, National Archives, Fort Worth, TX; "Applications for Headstones for US Military Veterans, 1925–1941," microfilm publication M1916, 134 rolls, ARC ID 596118, Records of the Office of the Quartermaster General, RG 92, National Archives, Washington, DC.

Jerry's injuries, Basilia as chief nurse: Dudley Early, "Admiral Jerry Steward, Legislator from Freestone, One of Few Men with a Navy Cross," *Waco Tribune Herald*, February 4, 1951.

Basilia added to roster: "Petition for Naturalization," no. 2353; Danner, *What a Way to Spend a War*.

Japanese uncertainty with nurses: Mary Rose Harrington, interview in *We All Came Home: Army and Navy Nurse POWs in WWII* (US Department of Defense, 1985), video, NTIS no. AVA14014VNB1.

Rape of Manila, Japanese attitude toward prisoners: John Pritchard and Sonia M. Zaide, eds., "International Military Tribunal for the Far East: Judgment of 12 November 1948," in *The Tokyo War Crimes Trial*, vol. 22 (New York: Garland, 1981).

Japanese arrival at Santa Scholastica: Bureau of Medicine and Surgery, "Interview with Bertha Evans"; Danner, *What a Way to Spend a War*; Bureau of Medicine and Surgery, "Oral History with Pharmacist's Mate Donald Tapscott."

Treatment of Guam nurses: Leona Jackson, "POW Notes," 1942, Office of Naval Records and Library.

Captain Davis had ordered through *the new guards looped barbed wire*: Bureau of Medicine and Surgery, "Interview with Bertha Evans"; Danner, *What a Way to Spend a War*; Kentner, "Daily Journal of Events."

Japanese military culture of theft: Sides, *Ghost Soldiers*.

Peg hiding ring in cold cream: Danner, *What a Way to Spend a War*; Bureau of Medicine and Surgery, "Interview with Margaret Nash."

Background of Edwin Wood: Bureau of Medicine and Surgery, "Interview with Margaret Nash"; "Mother Told Message Concerning Son," *Chicago Daily Tribune*, February 25, 1942; "Troth Announced of Anne Reynolds," *New York Times*, April 9, 1946; Edward N. Howard, oral history with Darlene Norman, Vigo County Public Library, Terre Haute, IN, December 18, 1980.

Quinine administration: Owsei Temkin and Elizabeth M. Ramsey, *Antimalarial Drugs: General Outline* (Washington, DC: National Research Council, 1944).

the army nurses were instructed: Redmond, *I Served on Baatan*.

She ordered her nurses to switch: Todd, "Nursing Under Fire"; Danner, *What a Way to Spend a War*; Johnson, "Laura Cobb."

Quinine's bitter taste: Temkin and Ramsey, *Antimalarial Drugs*.

5. Chin Up, Girls

Edwina menaced: Todd, "Nursing Under Fire."

Guard harassment, curfew: Danner, *What a Way to Spend a War.*

Work details and slaps: Danner, *What a Way to Spend a War*; Kentner, "Daily Journal of Events."

the force was far more severe: Giles, *Captive of the Rising Sun.*

Culture of violence in Japanese military: Tanaka, *Hidden Horrors.*

Volleyball game: Bureau of Medicine and Surgery, "Interview with Bertha Evans."

Removal of supplies and patients: Danner, *What a Way to Spend a War*; Kentner, "Daily Journal of Events."

February 14 was through *not even for nurses*: Jeffrey, *White Coolies*; Papers of Vivian Bullwinkel, coll. no. PR01216, Australian War Memorial.

Reservist escape and head count: Kentner, "Daily Journal of Events."

Peg marked for execution: Bureau of Medicine and Surgery, "Interview with Margaret Nash"; Danner, *What a Way to Spend a War.*

saw it was a warning: Todd, "Nursing Under Fire"; Kentner, "Daily Journal of Events."

Cobb's separation concerns, Dorothy's illness: Danner, *What a Way to Spend a War.*

likely contracted the virus: Charles P. Gerba and Denise Kennedy, "Enteric Virus Survival During Household Laundering and Impact of Disinfection with Sodium Hypochlorite," *Applied and Environmental Microbiology* 73, no. 14 (2007): 4425–4428.

Cobb was fearful through *new ways to breed*: Danner, *What a Way to Spend a War.*

Courtyard announcement and packing for transfer: Danner, *What a Way to Spend a War*; Todd, "Nursing Under Fire."

Davis's warning: Bureau of Medicine and Surgery, "Interview with Margaret Nash."

Cobb conceals records: Johnson, "Laura Cobb"; Danner, *What a Way to Spend a War.*

Of the 102 corpsmen: Author comparison of roster in Kentner, "Daily Journal of Events," January 2, 1942, with *US Navy Casualties Books, 1776–1941* and "State Summary of War Casualties from World War II for Navy, Marine Corps, and Coast Guard Personnel," Records of the Bureau of Naval Personnel, RG 24, both in National Archives, College Park, MD.

transporting thousands of prisoners: Maga, *Judgment at Tokyo*.

prisoners called them "hell ships" through eight of the eighteen hundred men survived: La Forte, Marcello, and Himmel, eds., *With Only the Will to Live*; Glusman, *Conduct Under Fire*.

All of the fifty-four corpsmen: Author comparison of roster and casualty lists.

6. Room 30A

Traveling through Manila: Danner, *What a Way to Spend a War*.

Santo Tomas description: Hartendorp, *Santo Tomas Story*.

Margaret Sherk was one of the have-nots: Sams, *Forbidden Family*.

Sherk's background: "Records of the Office of the Provost Marshal General, 1920–1975," no. 389, National Archives, Washington, DC; Sams, *Forbidden Family*.

Within weeks through *sip from the water fountain*: Hartendorp, *Santo Tomas Story*; Sams, *Forbidden Family*.

Camp bathrooms: Brines, *Until They Eat Stones*.

Trustworthy children: Vaughan, *Ordeal*.

Her anger depleted her sympathy: Sams, *Forbidden Family*.

Camp layout, leadership structure, and commander: Hartendorp, *Santo Tomas Story*.

Description of group photograph: Photograph courtesy of Bureau of Medicine and Surgery.

Description of 30A: Danner, *What a Way to Spend a War*; Sams, *Forbidden Family*.

Susie's health: Danner, *What a Way to Spend a War*; "California Death Index, 1940–1997," State of California Department of Health Services, Center for Health Statistics, Sacramento, CA.

Cobb as director of nursing: Johnson, "Laura Cobb"; Danner, *What a Way to Spend a War*.

Rumor of President Quezon's death: Hartendorp, *Santo Tomas Story*.

Quezon's exile: "Manuel Quezon, 65, Dies; Exiled Philippine Leader," *Mercury* (Pottstown, PA), August 2, 1944.

Bataan falls: Hartendorp, *Santo Tomas Story*; Danner, *What a Way to Spend a War*.

In the photo, a colonel sat: Description of photograph dated April 9, 1942, National Museum of the US Air Force.

King trusted the surrender: Yenne, *Imperial Japanese Army*.

Bataan Death March: Casey, *Engineers of the Southwest Pacific*.

new wave of inmates: Danner, *What a Way to Spend a War*.

Dorothy ached through *Roosevelt had addressed the nation*: Danner, *What a Way to Spend a War*; Hartendorp, *Santo Tomas Story*.

Execution of three escapees: Stevens, *Santo Tomas Internment Camp*.

Attack on ice cream vendor: Cates, *Drainpipe Diary*.

Peg forced to watch beating: Bureau of Medicine and Surgery, "Interview with Margaret Nash"; Cates, *Drainpipe Diary*.

Bathroom details and privacy methods: Danner, *What a Way to Spend a War*; Cates, *Drainpipe Diary*.

Food privileges: Danner, *What a Way to Spend a War*; Bureau of Medicine and Surgery, "Oral History with Dorothy Still Danner."

Susie's heart attack: Danner, *What a Way to Spend a War*.

Bertha's surgery: Bureau of Medicine and Surgery, "Interview with Bertha Evans."

And Edwina Todd became through *Edwina's bad moods*: Danner, *What a Way to Spend a War*; Norman, *We Band of Angels*.

Arrival of army nurses: Danner, *What a Way to Spend a War*; Norman, *We Band of Angels*; Monahan and Neidel-Greenlee, *All This Hell*.

"Gwendolyn! Gwendolyn!": Danner, *What a Way to Spend a War*.

Army women "quarantined": Danner, *What a Way to Spend a War*; Norman, *We Band of Angels*; Monahan and Neidel-Greenlee, *All This Hell*.

Army nurses take over, culture differences between army and navy nurses: Danner, *What a Way to Spend a War*.

Army nurses' relationship with other inmates: Wygle, *Surviving a Japanese P.O.W. Camp*; Sams, *Forbidden Family*.

7. Where Were You When We Needed Help?

Dorothy rested under a tree through *"Where were you"*: Danner, *What a Way to Spend a War.*

Nurses in Bataan: Redmond, *I Served on Baatan*; Norman, *We Band of Angels.*

Bombing of Hospital #1: Redmond, *I Served on Baatan.*

In the highest branches: Bureau of Medicine and Surgery, "Recollections of Ann Bernatitus."

evacuation orders came: Redmond, *I Served on Baatan*; Norman, *We Band of Angels*; Monahan and Neidel-Greenlee, *All This Hell.*

Ann Bernatitus received evacuation orders: Bureau of Medicine and Surgery, "Recollections of Ann Bernatitus."

these types of flashbacks: Danner, *What a Way to Spend a War.*

New commanders: Hartendorp, *Santo Tomas Story.*

Jail within a jail: Danner, *What a Way to Spend a War*; Hartendorp, *Santo Tomas Story.*

The commanders mostly focused: Stevens, *Santo Tomas Internment Camp.*

Shanties, loss of sexual function: Hartendorp, *Santo Tomas Story*; Danner, *What a Way to Spend a War.*

Christmas preparations and delivery concerns: Danner, *What a Way to Spend a War.*

Distribution of comfort kits: Hartendorp, *Santo Tomas Story*; Danner, *What a Way to Spend a War*; Cates, *Drainpipe Diary.*

Christmas in the camp through *momentary sense of calm*: Danner, *What a Way to Spend a War.*

Propaganda film: Hartendorp, *Santo Tomas Story*; Danner, *What a Way to Spend a War*; Cates, *Drainpipe Diary.*

Hollywood movie showing: Hartendorp, *Santo Tomas Story*; Cates, *Drainpipe Diary*; *The Feminine Touch*, directed by W. S. Van Dyke (1941; Burbank, CA: Warner Archive Collection, 2015), DVD.

The guards allowed through *"Forty-three and we'll be free"*: Danner, *What a Way to Spend a War*; Hartendorp, *Santo Tomas Story.*

8. Fed Up with the Way Things Have Been Going

Dorothy waiting: Danner, *What a Way to Spend a War*.

angry soldier had betrayed: Danner, *What a Way to Spend a War*; Hartendorp, *Santo Tomas Story*; Cates, *Drainpipe Diary*.

Difference between civilian and military captives: Butow, *Tojo*.

The men were well liked: Hartendorp, *Santo Tomas Story*.

"I can't begin to tell you": Danner, *What a Way to Spend a War*.

Removal of enlisted men: Hartendorp, *Santo Tomas Story*; Danner, *What a Way to Spend a War*.

sound of a sobbing woman: Cates, *Drainpipe Diary*.

Pleading with Kuroda, others ordered to register: Hartendorp, *Santo Tomas Story*; Danner, *What a Way to Spend a War*.

Descriptions of ailments at hospital: Cates, *Drainpipe Diary*.

Dispute over housing: Danner, *What a Way to Spend a War*; Hartendorp, *Santo Tomas Story*.

A strike had potential through *compromise with the army nurses*: Danner, *What a Way to Spend a War*.

Housing deal reached: Hartendorp, *Santo Tomas Story*.

Gwendolyn admits to using Dorothy: Danner, *What a Way to Spend a War*.

Nurses' coping mechanisms: Danner, *What a Way to Spend a War*; "Reported Missing," *Chicago Daily Tribune*, July 19, 1942; Bureau of Medicine and Surgery, "Interview with Bertha Evans."

Expectant mothers: Hartendorp, *Santo Tomas Story*; Cates, *Drainpipe Diary*.

Return of the enlisted men: Hartendorp, *Santo Tomas Story*; Stevens, *Santo Tomas Internment Camp*.

9. They Will Suffocate!

Worry about typhoons: Cates, *Drainpipe Diary*.

A disturbance was indeed through *intercamp communication possible*: Hartendorp, *Santo Tomas Story*; Butow, *Tojo*.

Commander's announcement: Danner, *What a Way to Spend a War*; Hartendorp, *Santo Tomas Story*.

Fears of leaving: Danner, *What a Way to Spend a War*; Hartendorp, *Santo Tomas Story*; Cates, *Drainpipe Diary*.

Only two hundred men volunteered through *six hundred able-bodied men*: Hartendorp, *Santo Tomas Story*; Cates, *Drainpipe Diary*.

Mary Rose finds Dorothy: Danner, *What a Way to Spend a War*.

Leach had asked: Bureau of Medicine and Surgery, "Interview with Bertha Evans."

Cobb decides each nurse must answer: Johnson, "Laura Cobb."

Decision to leave: Danner, *What a Way to Spend a War*.

It was only 5:00 AM: Cates, *Drainpipe Diary*.

Margaret Sherk's unhappiness: Sams, *Forbidden Family*.

Turning over luggage: Danner, *What a Way to Spend a War*; Bureau of Medicine and Surgery, "Oral History with Dorothy Still Danner."

Dorothy tried to look forward through *Anchors Aweigh*: Danner, *What a Way to Spend a War*; Bureau of Medicine and Surgery, "Interview with Mary Rose Harrington."

Arriving at station, seeing boxcars: Danner, *What a Way to Spend a War*; Bureau of Medicine and Surgery, "Oral History with Dorothy Still Danner"; Bureau of Medicine and Surgery, "Interview with Mary Rose Harrington."

Nash's reaction: Bureau of Medicine and Surgery, "Interview with Margaret Nash."

Cobb's response: Danner, *What a Way to Spend a War*; Bureau of Medicine and Surgery, "Interview with Mary Rose Harrington."

Women divided, boxcar doors shut: Danner, *What a Way to Spend a War*; Bureau of Medicine and Surgery, "Oral History with Dorothy Still Danner"; Bureau of Medicine and Surgery, "Interview with Mary Rose Harrington."

The doors remained locked through *water bottles were soon empty*: Danner, *What a Way to Spend a War*.

Using hat for fan: Bureau of Medicine and Surgery, "Interview with Mary Rose Harrington."

Dorothy's thoughts on the journey: Danner, *What a Way to Spend a War*.

10. Take Them Outside

Men forced to walk, women in truck: Danner, *What a Way to Spend a War*.

The soldier assigned to the truck through *improved immediately*: Bureau of Medicine and Surgery, "Interview with Mary Rose Harrington."

Dorothy's first impression of camp: Bureau of Medicine and Surgery, "Oral History with Dorothy Still Danner"; Danner, *What a Way to Spend a War*.

Served sake, photo taken: Bureau of Medicine and Surgery, "Interview with Bertha Evans."

Peg Nash and propaganda photos: Bureau of Medicine and Surgery, "Interview with Margaret Nash"; "Lee Park Nurse Pictured at Jap Prison Camp," *Wilkes-Barre Record*, December 27, 1944.

Descriptions of camp in US newspapers: "Lee Park Nurse Held Prisoner by Japanese," *Wilkes-Barre Record*, September 29, 1942.

Juanita Redmond: US Army Signal Corps, "I Was There Corregidor (1943)" (film), *Army-Navy Screen Magazine* 5 (1943).

Forced to sleep on baseball diamond: Henderson, *Rescue at Los Baños*.

Malaria concerns, dormitory feels private: Bureau of Medicine and Surgery, "Oral History with Dorothy Still Danner."

Chicken hunt: Bureau of Medicine and Surgery, "Interview with Mary Rose Harrington"; Peg Nash, interview in *We All Came Home*, video.

Infirmary description: Danner, *What a Way to Spend a War*; Bureau of Medicine and Surgery, "Oral History with Dorothy Still Danner."

Stripped hospital: Bureau of Medicine and Surgery, "Interview with Bertha Evans"; Bureau of Medicine and Surgery, "Oral History with Dorothy Still Danner"; Danner, *What a Way to Spend a War*; Bureau of Medicine and Surgery, "Interview with Margaret Nash"; Todd, "Nursing Under Fire."

Bedrolls and jusi: Todd, "Nursing Under Fire."

Uniforms and bandages: Bureau of Medicine and Surgery, "Interview with Mary Rose Harrington"; Danner, *What a Way to Spend a War*.

Pharmaceutical solutions: Todd, "Nursing Under Fire."

Negotiating for supplies: Danner, *What a Way to Spend a War*; Bureau of Medicine and Surgery, "Oral History with Dorothy Still Danner."

Resistance through radios: Sams, *Forbidden Family*; Bureau of Medicine and Surgery, "Interview with Mary Rose Harrington."

Repatriation of Dr. Leach: Danner, *What a Way to Spend a War*; Bureau of Medicine and Surgery, "Oral History with Dorothy Still Danner."

Background on Dr. Dana Nance: State of Tennessee, Delayed Certificate of Birth, 359917, Tennessee State Library and Archives, Nashville, TN; "Passport Applications for Travel to China, 1906–1925," box 4421, vol. 9, National Archives, Washington, DC.

The nurses were excited through *guards' problems did not interest the inmates*: Danner, *What a Way to Spend a War*; Bureau of Medicine and Surgery, "Interview with Mary Rose Harrington"; Bureau of Medicine and Surgery, "Interview with Margaret Nash."

11. I Am Ashamed of You

Prepping for class, need for orderlies: Danner, *What a Way to Spend a War*; Bureau of Medicine and Surgery, "Oral History with Dorothy Still Danner."

Clinic demands: Bureau of Medicine and Surgery, "Interview with Margaret Nash."

Training orderlies: Danner, *What a Way to Spend a War*; Bureau of Medicine and Surgery, "Oral History with Dorothy Still Danner."

Navy Hospital Corps handbook and Dorothy's fascination with its procedures: US Navy, *Handbook of the Hospital Corps*; Danner, *What a Way to Spend a War*.

Extra orderlies in class: Danner, *What a Way to Spend a War*.

Thomas Terrill background: US Census 1940, Queens, NY, roll m-t0627-02744, p. 7A, enumeration district 41-1239; State of California Divorce Index, 1966, Center for Health Statistics, California Department of Health Services, Sacramento, CA.

Flight routes in 1941: "1941 Arrival to La Guardia Field, New York, New York," microfilm serial T715 (1897–1957), microfilm 6538, line 5, p. 66C; "1941 Arrival to New York, New York," microfilm serial T715

(1897–1957), microfilm 6543, line 15, p. 5; "Passenger & Crew Manifests of Airplanes Arriving at Baltimore, Maryland," 1787–2004, NAI no. 2642537, all in Records of the Immigration and Naturalization Service, RG 85, National Archives, Washington, DC.

Thomas's arrival in Manila: Outward Manifest, November 2, 1941, Honolulu, "List of Persons on American Owned Airplanes," 1787–2004, NAI no. 2642537, Records of the Immigration and Naturalization Service, RG 85, National Archives, Washington DC.

Thomas's physical appearance: *The Big T of 1932* (Pasadena, CA: California Institute of Technology, 1932), student yearbook.

attended the same junior college: *Campus* (Pasadena, CA: Pasadena Junior College, 1933), student yearbook.

Stargazing: Danner, *What a Way to Spend a War.*

Peg's friend: Danner, *What a Way to Spend a War.*

Goldia and Robert Merrill: Chuck Mueller, "Imprisoned Woman Finds Way to Help," *San Bernardino County Sun*, October 10, 1993; Robert Merrill service record, Electronic Army Serial Number Merged File, 1938–1946, ARC 1263923, "World War II Army Enlistment Records," RG 64, National Archives, Washington, DC; Robert Merrill imprisonment record, "World War II Prisoners of War Data File, 12/7/1941–11/19/1946," NAI no. 1263907, RG 389, National Archives, Washington, DC.

Mary Rose and T. Page Nelson: Marylou Tousignant and Rich Pedroncelli, "Prisoners of War, Prisoners of Love," *Washington Post*, April 13, 1995; Bart Barnes, "Treasury Official T. Page Nelson Sr. Dies at 80," *Washington Post*, March 17, 1999; "Draft Registration Cards for District of Columbia, 10/16/1940–03/31/1947," RG 147, box 169, National Archives, St. Louis, MO.

Tensions at the hospital, treatment of scabies: Danner, *What a Way to Spend a War*; US Navy, *Handbook of the Hospital Corps.*

Dorothy stiffened through *eat a papaya*: Danner, *What a Way to Spend a War.*

Dysentery treatment: Lenna F. Cooper, Edith M. Barber, and Helen S. Mitchell, *Nutrition in Health and Disease* (Philadelphia: J. B. Lippincott, 1930).

Cobb ends conflict, Dorothy fumes, Thomas comforts her with haircut, and
    Dorothy's surgery: Danner, *What a Way to Spend a War*.
Hydrocele: Clarence Rutherford O'Crowley and Jacob Herzlich, "Hydro-
    cele: Its Relationship to Hernia," *American Journal of Surgery* 66, no. 2
    (1944): 157–60.
Post-healing boredom: Danner, *What a Way to Spend a War*.
Worsening conditions at Santo Tomas: Cates, *Drainpipe Diary*; Brines, *Until
    They Eat Stones*.
Comfort kits: Hartendorp, *Santo Tomas Story*; Cates, *Drainpipe Diary*;
    Vaughan, *Ordeal*.
Christmas at Los Baños and Peg Nash in hospital: Danner, *What a Way to
    Spend a War*; Bureau of Medicine and Surgery, "Interview with Mar-
    garet Nash."

12. We Might Not Come Out of This Alive

Water and sanitation concerns: Arthur, *Deliverance at Los Baños*; Bureau of
    Medicine and Surgery, "Interview with Bertha Evans."
Family reunion: Hartendorp, *Santo Tomas Story*; Cates, *Drainpipe Diary*;
    Cogan, *Captured*.
mailing instructions were confusing: Giles, *Captive of the Rising Sun*.
Dorothy's letter home: Dorothy Still, letter to William and Arissa Still, August
    9, 1943, courtesy of Bureau of Medicine and Surgery.
Coded messages: Giles, *Captive of the Rising Sun*.
Dorothy heard her name called through *never eating outside again*: Danner,
    What a Way to Spend a War.
Bertha at the new table: Bureau of Medicine and Surgery, "Interview with
    Bertha Evans."
Allied forces were advancing: MacArthur, *Reminiscences*.
part of a new operation: Morton, *War in the Pacific*.
Southern Philippines looking possible: MacArthur, *Reports of General
    MacArthur*.
Margaret Sherk's letters to husband, decision to move to Los Baños: Sams,
    Forbidden Family.

transfer of more than five hundred prisoners: Arthur, *Deliverance at Los Baños*; Hartendorp, *Santo Tomas Story*.

Margaret reunites with Gerald, reacts to new camp: Sams, *Forbidden Family*.

Transfer of undesirable inmates: Danner, *What a Way to Spend a War*; Bureau of Medicine and Surgery, "Interview with Bertha Evans."

The infirmary was soon at capacity: Monahan and Neidel-Greenlee, *All This Hell*.

Vegetable thefts, Dana's accusations, Dorothy and Eldene move to barracks: Danner, *What a Way to Spend a War*.

13. I Have Returned

"Senile" commander, Konishi arrives, inmates devastated: Cogan, *Captured*; Arthur, *Deliverance at Los Baños*; Hartendorp, *Santo Tomas Story*; Danner, *What a Way to Spend a War*.

Konishi's taunts: Danner, *What a Way to Spend a War*.

Konishi's physical appearance and background: Cogan, *Captured*; Arthur, *Deliverance at Los Baños*; Hartendorp, *Santo Tomas Story*; Danner, *What a Way to Spend a War*.

Japanese racism: Tanaka, *Hidden Horrors*.

Japan's military losses: Owens, *Eye-Deep in Hell*.

Cutting of rations: Danner, *What a Way to Spend a War*.

One inmate thought confiscating money: Peter and Ethel Chapman, *Escape to the Hills*.

Bertha sees US plane: Bureau of Medicine and Surgery, "Interview with Bertha Evans."

US major learns of Los Baños: Henderson, *Rescue at Los Baños*.

no longer had a menstrual cycle: Danner, *What a Way to Spend a War*.

Incontinence: Todd, "Nursing Under Fire."

Twelve-hour shifts: Johnson, "Laura Cobb."

Trembling and falling: Todd, "Nursing Under Fire"; Danner, *What a Way to Spend a War*.

Civilian lack of appreciation: Danner, *What a Way to Spend a War*; Grace Nash, *That We Might Live*.

Irving Posner background: "US Passport Applications, Hawaii, Puerto Rico
    and Philippines, 1907–1925," vol. 30, National Archives, Washington,
    DC.
Posner dies, Dana offers comfort: Stevens, *Santo Tomas Internment Camp*;
    Arthur, *Deliverance at Los Baños*.
Life expectancy and deaths of other inmates: R. D. Grove and A. M. Hetzel,
    Vital Statistics Rates in the United States, 1940–1960 (Washington, DC:
    US Government Printing Office, 1968); Danner, *What a Way to Spend a
    War*; "World War II and Korean Conflict Veterans Interred Overseas,"
    s.v. "Grace McGuire," National Archives, Washington, DC.
Burt Fonger's death: "World War II and Korean Conflict Veterans Interred
    Overseas," s.v. "Burton Fonger," National Archives, Washington, DC;
    Arthur, *Deliverance at Los Baños*; Danner, *What a Way to Spend a War*.
Fonger's orchestra attempts and burial, commander's Christmas promise:
    Grace Nash, *That We Might Live*.
Inmates were coming in droves: Todd, "Nursing Under Fire."

14. Do the Best You Can

Violent death from beriberi: Danner, *What a Way to Spend a War*; Ralph
    Hibbs, "Beriberi in Japanese Prison Camp," *Annals of Internal Medicine*
    25 (1946): 270–282; US War Department, *Annual Report of the Secre-
    tary of War*, vol. 2, pt. 2 (Washington, DC: US Government Printing
    Office, 1901).
Broken collarbone: T. W. McGarry, "Prisoners of Japanese Liberate the
    Memory of Raid on Los Banos," *Los Angeles Times*, May 14, 1985.
Slashed leg: Dorothy Still, war crimes statement, September 10, 1945, declas-
    sified NND 775011, National Archives, Washington, DC.
Slapping of inmate: Arthur, *Deliverance at Los Baños*.
Woman forced to bow repeatedly: Henderson, *Rescue at Los Baños*.
Fights between inmates: Arthur, *Deliverance at Los Baños*; Bryant, *The Sun
    Was Darkened*.
Camp bully: Grace Nash, *That We Might Live*.

Cats as food: Bureau of Medicine and Surgery, "Interview with Mary Rose Harrington."

Death to Poochie: Danner, *What a Way to Spend a War*; McGarry, "Prisoners of Japanese"; Arthur, *Deliverance at Los Baños*.

Deaths from malnutrition: Danner, *What a Way to Spend a War*; Arthur, *Deliverance at Los Baños*.

Eating leaves and insects: Rubens, *Bread and Rice*.

Camp illness, loss of homemade supplies: Danner, *What a Way to Spend a War*; Beaber, *Deliverance!*

Chief Nurse Cobb encouraged through *food donation from the Vatican*: Danner, *What a Way to Spend a War*.

Margaret Sherk's operation and tuberculosis: Sams, *Forbidden Family*; A. K. Sharma, "Abdominal Tuberculosis of the Gastrointestinal Tract: Revisited." *World Journal of Gastroenterology* 20, no. 40 (2014): 14831–14840.

Palawan massacre: Rufus W. Smith, oral history with George Burlage, University of North Texas Oral History Program, 1989; Neil Boister and Robert Cryer, eds., *Documents on the Tokyo International Military Tribunal: Charter, Indictment and Judgments* (New York: Oxford University Press, 2008); Glenn McDole, oral history with William Alexander, National Museum of the Pacific War, 1996; "Japanese Atrocities: Report of the Department of State," *Department of State Bulletin* 13, no. 321 (1945).

Physical appearance of Los Baños inmates: Author analysis of Bureau of Medicine and Surgery photographs and US Army Signal Corps archival film footage.

Selling of jewelry for fruit: Grace Nash, *That We Might Live*.

Dorothy's Christmas: Danner, *What a Way to Spend a War*.

In-depth food conversations: Bureau of Medicine and Surgery, "Interview with Margaret Nash"; Grace Nash, interview in *We All Came Home*, video.

the Japanese abandoned organized resistance: Owens, *Eye-Deep in Hell*.

liquidated the Baguio prison camp: Hind, *Spirits Unbroken*.

Konishi refused to accept: Sams, *Forbidden Family*.

15. 'Tis You, 'Tis You Must Go and I Must Bide

Hugh Williams background: "Hugh Hoskyn [*sic*] Williams," Auckland
   Museum War Memorial Online, accessed January 4, 2019, www.auckland
   museum.com/war-memorial/online-cenotaph/record/C129744.

Williams's kindness to children: Danner, *What a Way to Spend a War*; Grace
   Nash, *That We Might Live*.

Williams's relationship with Cobb: Danner, *What a Way to Spend a War*.

his last can of condensed milk: Danner, *What a Way to Spend a War*; Grace
   Nash, *That We Might Live*.

Dorothy sleeping through baby's birth: Bureau of Medicine and Surgery,
   "Interview with Margaret Nash"; Danner, *What a Way to Spend a War*.

Eldene wakes Dorothy: Danner, *What a Way to Spend a War*.

Sneaking outside, threat of retribution: Danner, *What a Way to Spend a
   War*; Bureau of Medicine and Surgery, "Oral History with Dorothy Still
   Danner."

the paperwork he wanted to process: Arthur, *Deliverance at Los Baños*.

Looting, flag ceremony: Danner, *What a Way to Spend a War*; Arthur, *Deliverance at Los Baños*; Grace Nash, *That We Might Live*.

The administrative committee announced new rules: Danner, *What a Way
   to Spend a War*; Arthur, *Deliverance at Los Baños*.

prisoners who were formerly radio operators through *"We are here to protect
   you"*: Danner, *What a Way to Spend a War*; Arthur, *Deliverance at
   Los Baños*; Grace Nash, *That We Might Live*: Bureau of Medicine and
   Surgery, "Oral History with Dorothy Still Danner."

Howard Hell background and death: "Remembering Howard Hell," *MSM
   Alumnus* (MSM-UMR Alumni Association), Summer 1996; American
   Foreign Service, Report of the Death of an American Citizen, no. 311B.113,
   April 16, 1946; "Candidates for Degrees," *Rolla Herald*, June 1, 1933;
   Round About, *Gasconade County Republican* (Owenville, MO) February
   4, 1943; "Hungry Days in Enemy Prison Camp Described," *Rolla Herald*,
   September 20, 1945; "Cuba Review," *Rolla Herald*, July 24, 1941; Bureau
   of Medicine and Surgery, "Oral History with Dorothy Still Danner."

16. Roll Out the Barrel

Shot heard: Danner, *What a Way to Spend a War*; Bureau of Medicine and Surgery, "Oral History with Dorothy Still Danner."

An inmate was slumped on the ground: "Summary Execution Protested," Department of State bulletin, September 9, 1945, in *Congressional Record*, 79th Cong., 1st sess., appendix 91, pt. 12, A3788.

George Louis shot returning to camp: Danner, *What a Way to Spend a War*; Bureau of Medicine and Surgery, "Oral History with Dorothy Still Danner."

The committee members protested: Danner, *What a Way to Spend a War*; Bureau of Medicine and Surgery, "Oral History with Dorothy Still Danner"; Arthur, *Deliverance at Los Baños*.

George Louis executed: Danner, *What a Way to Spend a War*; Bureau of Medicine and Surgery, "Oral History with Dorothy Still Danner"; Lucas, *Prisoners of Santo Tomas*; Still, war crimes statement.

Handling of George's body: Danner, *What a Way to Spend a War*; Bureau of Medicine and Surgery, "Oral History with Dorothy Still Danner."

Cabanatuan deaths: "Historical Report: US Casualties and Burials at Cabanatuan POW Camp #1," Defense POW/MIA Accounting Agency, May 8, 2017, www.dpaa.mil/Portals/85/Documents/Reports/U.S.Casualties _Burials_Cabanatuan_POWCamp1.pdf?ver=2017-05-08-162357-013.

Robert Lapham background and guerrilla work: Lapham and Norling, *Lapham's Raiders*.

Lieutenant Colonel Henry Mucci: Robert McG. Thomas Jr. "Henry A. Mucci Dies at 88. Rescued Survivors of Bataan," *New York Times*, April 24, 1997.

"It's the Americans": Arthur Veysey, "Rangers Kill 532 Japs; Take Camp in Half Hour," *Chicago Tribune*, February 2, 1945.

Raid on Cabanatuan: Sides, *Ghost Soldiers*; "Raid Enemy Prison Camp in Philippines," *Mount Pleasant (IA) News*, February 1, 1945; "Writer Tells How Line of Captives Came Back," *Daily Chronicle* (DeKalb, IL), February 1, 1945; "Rangers Execute Daring Attack to Free Allies," *Rocky*

Mount (NC) Telegram, February 1, 1945; Dean Schedler, "Americans Joyous," *Rocky Mount Telegram*, February 1, 1945.

Americans loved liberation stories: "4,500 Civilians in Manila Wait Liberation," *Chicago Daily Tribune*, February 3, 1945.

"and already looked like new men": "Manila to Fall in Hours, W-G-N Reporter Says," *Chicago Daily Tribune*, February 3, 1945.

Newspapers dealing with Japanese atrocities: Charles Jensen, "Yes, the Japs Pay Prisoners—3 Cents a Day!" *Chicago Daily Tribune*, February 4, 1945.

the "Cabanatuan Shuffle": Hibbs, "Beriberi in Japanese Prison Camp."

Jerry Steward at Cabanatuan: Early, "Admiral Jerry Steward."

Liberation of Santo Tomas: Cates, *Drainpipe Diary*; Hartendorp, *Santo Tomas Story*; Ray Perez, "4 Decades Later, Civilian POWs Reunite to Remember," *Los Angeles Times*, February 14, 1986; Stevens, *Santo Tomas Internment Camp*.

Rape of Manila: US Army Signal Corps, archival film footage, September 18, 1947, rec. no. 1964708, 330-DVIC-24, National Archives, Washington, DC; US Army Signal Corps, archival film footage, February 15, 1945, rec. no. 23569, 111-ADC-9804, National Archives, Washington, DC.

17. Today We Either Live or Die

Dorothy stumbled through the ward: Danner, *What a Way to Spend a War*; Todd, "Nursing Under Fire."

Cobb encouraging but fading: Danner, *What a Way to Spend a War*.

Too tired to fight, envy for the dead: Danner, *What a Way to Spend a War*; Bureau of Medicine and Surgery, "Oral History with Dorothy Still Danner."

Machine guns, rumors of massacre: Johnson, "Laura Cobb"; Danner, *What a Way to Spend a War*; Bureau of Medicine and Surgery, "Interview with Mary Rose Harrington"; Carter and Mueller, *Combat Chronology*.

Injured baby: Danner, *What a Way to Spend a War*; Todd, "Nursing Under Fire."

Dorothy's night shift through *swayed toward the ground*: Danner, *What a Way to Spend a War*; Bureau of Medicine and Surgery, "Oral History with Dorothy Still Danner."

Peg Nash went to the window: Bureau of Medicine and Surgery, "Interview with Margaret Nash."

Guerrillas hunt guards, plan of attack: Todd, "Nursing Under Fire"; Bureau of Medicine and Surgery, "Oral History with Dorothy Still Danner"; Steve Ellis, "Los Baños' Freedom Day," *V.F.W. Magazine*, February 1979.

Inmates' bizarre behavior: Bob Wheeler and Margaret Squires, interview in *Rescue at Dawn: The Los Baños Raid*, A&E Television Networks, July 17, 2008.

Amtracs: David Sullens, "Amtracs Unique to Marines," *Galveston Daily News*, October 25, 1989; Jeter Allen Isely and Phillip Axtell Crowl, *The U.S. Marines and Amphibious War: Its Theory and Its Practice in the Pacific* (Princeton, NJ: Princeton University Press, 1951); Flanagan, *The Los Baños Raid*.

A line of more than fifty through *What did they do to you?*: Danner, *What a Way to Spend a War*; Charlie Sass, interview in *Rescue at Dawn*, A&E.

Soldiers liberate the infirmary: Danner, *What a Way to Spend a War*; Bureau of Medicine and Surgery, "Oral History with Dorothy Still Danner."

Peg asks for food: Peg Nash, interview in *We All Came Home*, video.

Peg and Susie loaded into Jeep: Danner, *What a Way to Spend a War*; Todd, "Nursing Under Fire"; Johnson, "Laura Cobb"; Bureau of Medicine and Surgery, "Interview with Margaret Nash."

inmates were packing their belongings: Danner, *What a Way to Spend a War*; Bureau of Medicine and Surgery, "Oral History with Dorothy Still Danner."

Soldiers used military lingo: Sass, interview in *Rescue at Dawn*, A&E.

looked sadly at a toy box: Jim Holzem, interview in *Rescue at Dawn*, A&E.

Dorothy gives up: Danner, *What a Way to Spend a War*.

eight thousand Japanese soldiers: Todd, "Nursing Under Fire."

the "Impatient Virgin": Flanagan, *The Los Baños Raid*; *Rescue at Dawn*, A&E.

stragglers had to walk through *She passed the tin*: Danner, *What a Way to Spend a War*; Bureau of Medicine and Surgery, "Oral History with Dorothy Still Danner"; Bureau of Medicine and Surgery, "Interview with Bertha Evans"; Johnson, "Laura Cobb"; Bureau of Medicine and Surgery, "Interview with Margaret Nash"; Bureau of Medicine and Surgery, "Interview with Mary Rose Harrington"; McGarry, "Prisoners of Japanese."

Peg, Susie, Mary Rose, and Page depart: Bureau of Medicine and Surgery, "Interview with Margaret Nash"; Bureau of Medicine and Surgery, "Interview with Mary Rose Harrington."

Dorothy, Eldene, and Bertha through *until the end*: Danner, *What a Way to Spend a War*; Bureau of Medicine and Surgery, "Oral History with Dorothy Still Danner"; photograph of Eldene and Dorothy nursing on top of amtrac supplied by Bureau of Medicine and Surgery.

In the coming days through *an order was an order*: Jintaro Ishida, *The Remains of War: Apology and Forgiveness* (Guilford, CT: Lyons Press, 2002); "Chinese Tell of Massacre by Japanese," *Valley Morning Star* (Harlingen, TX), November 13, 1945; Pritchard and Zaide, eds., "International Military Tribunal for the Far East."

18. Don't Worry Anymore About Me

Second staging area: Danner, *What a Way to Spend a War*; Bureau of Medicine and Surgery, "Oral History with Dorothy Still Danner"; US Army Signal Corps, archival film footage, February 23, 1945, no. 4854, National Archives, Washington, DC; "Register of Citizen Arrivals (1943–1947) and Alien Arrivals (1936–1949) by Aircraft at San Francisco, California," NAI no. 4490795, RG 85, National Archives, Washington, DC.

Letters home: Danner, *What a Way to Spend a War*; Dorothy Still, letter to Arissa and William Still, February 24, 1945, courtesy of Bureau of Medicine and Surgery.

Food line, discarded meat: US Army Signal Corps, archival film footage, February 23, 1945; Danner, *What a Way to Spend a War*.

Excitement over tin cans: Sams, *Forbidden Family*.

They were concentration camp survivors: MacArthur, *Reminiscences*.

Bob Sherk: Sams, *Forbidden Family*; "Register, World War II Dead Interred in American Military Cemeteries on Foreign Soil and World War II and

Korea Missing or Lost or Buried at Sea," RG 389, National Archives, Washington, DC; "Commonwealth of Virginia Marriage Records, 1934–2014," no. 2230, Department of Health, Richmond, VA.

Grace Nash whispered with an intelligence corps officer: Grace Nash, *That We Might Live.*

Nursing at Bilibid: Danner, *What a Way to Spend a War*; Johnson, "Laura Cobb"; Todd, "Nursing Under Fire."

Jerry Steward looking for Basilia: Early, "Admiral Jerry Steward."

Jerry's weight: "Long Hard Fight Ahead Is Fighter's Opinion," *Pampa (TX) Daily News*, May 17, 1945.

Admiral Kinkaid greets the nurses: Bureau of Medicine and Surgery photo archives, nos. 09-8156-11 and 09-8156-12; Danner, *What a Way to Spend a War*; Bureau of Medicine and Surgery, "Oral History with Dorothy Still Danner"; Bureau of Medicine and Surgery, "Interview with Mary Rose Harrington."

Back pay: Danner, *What a Way to Spend a War*; Bureau of Medicine and Surgery, "Interview with Mary Rose Harrington"; Laura Cobb personnel file, courtesy of Bureau of Medicine and Surgery.

She was approached by a lieutenant: Danner, *What a Way to Spend a War.*

Luncheon: Danner, *What a Way to Spend a War*; Bureau of Medicine and Surgery, "Oral History with Dorothy Still Danner"; Bureau of Medicine and Surgery, "Interview with Mary Rose Harrington"; Bureau of Medicine and Surgery photo archives, nos. 09-8156-56, 09-8156-57, 09-8156-58, 09-8156-59, 09-8156-60, and 09-8156-61.

Dorothy chewed her filet mignon: Danner, *What a Way to Spend a War*; Bureau of Medicine and Surgery, "Interview with Mary Rose Harrington"; Bureau of Medicine and Surgery, "Oral History with Dorothy Still Danner."

Treats, alcohol prohibition: Bureau of Medicine and Surgery, "Interview with Margaret Nash"; Danner, *What a Way to Spend a War*; Bureau of Medicine and Surgery, "Interview with Mary Rose Harrington"; Bureau of Medicine and Surgery, "Oral History with Dorothy Still Danner"; Bureau of Medicine and Surgery, "Interview with Bertha Evans."

transport to Guam: Danner, *What a Way to Spend a War*; Bureau of Medicine and Surgery, "Oral History with Dorothy Still Danner"; Bureau of Medicine and Surgery, "Interview with Mary Rose Harrington."

Cobb and Nash want to return: "Lieut. Laura Cobb wants to go back," *Chillicothe Constitution Tribune*, March 13, 1945; "Rescued Nurses Request Action," *Fresno Bee*, March 6, 1945.

Publicity photos: Bureau of Medicine and Surgery photo archives, nos. 09-8156-33, 09-8156-53, and 09-8156-54.

the women underwent medical examinations: Bureau of Medicine and Surgery, "Interview with Margaret Nash."

Parade for Peg: Bureau of Medicine and Surgery, "Interview with Margaret Nash"; "5,000 Welcome Margaret Nash," *Wilkes-Barre Record*, March 27, 1945.

Civilians' comments, Dorothy's emotions: Danner, *What a Way to Spend a War*.

Ferdinand Berley's emotional response: Bureau of Medicine and Surgery, "Oral History with Ferdinand Berley."

Peg reunites with, ends relationship with Edwin: "Engaged to Marry," *New York Times*, April 9, 1946; "The Saga of Margaret Nash, WWII POW" (oral history), 1992, Women in Military Service to America Memorial Foundation, Arlington, VA.

Post-traumatic stress disorder: Giles, *Captive of the Rising Sun*.

Feeling useless: Danner, *What a Way to Spend a War*.

Postwar events: Bureau of Medicine and Surgery, "Oral History with Dorothy Still Danner"; Danner, *What a Way to Spend a War*.

Dorothy and the psychiatrist: Author interview with Dan Danner, January 8, 2018.

Epilogue: I Hear You

Henry Carpenter's realization: Flanagan, *The Los Baños Raid*; "Passenger Lists of Vessels Arriving at San Pedro/Wilmington/Los Angeles, California," NAI no. 4486355, RG 85, National Archives, Washington, DC.

Konishi interrogation: Interrogation report, November 28, 1945, Department of Defense, Department of the Army, Civilian Affairs Division,

War Crimes Branch, rec. no. 1754218, National Archives, Washington, DC; Records of the Law Division, Supreme Commander for the
Allied Powers, Legal Section, Manila Branch, November 1945 to 1949,
rec. no. 350136, National Archives, Washington, DC.

Konishi's sentence: "Fourth Supplement to the Synopses of National Trials,"
United Nations War Crimes Commission, C.255, April 30, 1947, Library
of Congress, Washington, DC.

lawyers claiming he had tuberculosis: "Attorneys Clash of Postponement in
Jap War Trial," *Harrisburg (PA) Telegraph*, November 23, 1946.

Konishi executed: Ginn, *Sugamo Prison*.

POW mortality: Bernard M. Cohen and Maurice Z. Cooper, *A Follow-Up
Study of World War II Prisoners of War* (Washington, DC: US Government Printing Office, 1954); Gary K. Reynolds, "US Prisoners of War
and Civilian American Citizens Captured and Interned by the Japanese
in World War II," Congressional Research Service, December 17, 2002.

Filipino loss of life: "Research Starters: Worldwide Deaths in World War II,"
National World War II Museum official website, accessed January 4, 2019,
www.nationalww2museum.org/students-teachers/student-resources
/research-starters/research-starters-worldwide-deaths-world-war.

Ann: Bureau of Medicine and Surgery, "Recollections of Ann Bernatitus";
Jan K. Herman, "In Memoriam: Capt. Ann Bernatitus, NC, USN (Ret),"
Navy Medicine 94, no. 3 (2003): 30.

Dana: Personals, *Deke Quarterly* 73, no. 4 (1955): 150; Perez, "4 Decades
Later"; Death Record 411-44-4051, Death Master List, US Social Security
Administration.

Gwendolyn: American Foreign Service, Report of the Death of an American
Citizen, May 11, 1960, Department of State, RG 59, entry 205, box 386,
National Archives, Washington, DC.

Jerry and Basilia: "Applications for Headstones for US Military Veterans,"
Records of the Office of the Quartermaster General; Death Record
460-52-8805, Death Master List, US Social Security Administration;
"Petitions for Naturalization," Records of District Courts of the United
States; Certificate of Death 67825 (November 28, 1965), "Texas Death
Certificates, 1903–1982," Texas Department of State Services, Austin, TX;

Early, "Admiral Jerry Steward"; "Jerry Steward," Legislative Reference Library of Texas, accessed January 4, 2019, https://lrl.texas.gov/mobile /memberDisplay.cfm?memberID=1422.

Susie: "Death Takes Susie Pitcher," *Des Moines Tribune*, January 3, 1951.

Helen: "Crash Kills Two Women," *Times* (San Mateo, CA), August 26, 1974; "Crash Kills Three," *Santa Cruz Sentinel*, August 26, 1974.

Cobb: Johnson, "Laura Cobb"; Cobb personnel file, courtesy of Bureau of Medicine and Surgery.

Peg: Personals, *Wilkes-Barre Times Leader*, August 4 & 31, 1948; Bureau of Medicine and Surgery, "Interview with Margaret Nash."

Bertha: "Five Military Nurses Coming to Convention," *Daily Capital Journal* (Salem, OR), October 21, 1954; Oregon Death Index, no. 01-25107, Oregon State Archives, Salem, OR.

Edwina: "Navy Nurse Senior Corps Member Retires," *United States Navy Medical Newsletter* 48, no. 8 (1966): 21; California Death Index, no. 561541149, State of California Department of Health Services, Center for Health Statistics, Sacramento, CA.

Mary Chapman: "Reported Missing," *Chicago Daily Tribune*, July 19, 1942; "Navy Nurse Home from Jap Prison," *Monitor* (McAllen, TX), June 7, 1945; Robert Widrich, "A Heroine," *Chicago Daily Tribune*, November 18, 1968; Death Record 527-52-0813, Death Master List, US Social Security Administration.

Goldia: "Navy Nurses to Be Decorated for Heroic Acts," *Eau Claire Leader*, September 5, 1945; "Passenger Lists of Vessels Arriving at San Pedro/ Wilmington/Los Angeles, California," NAI no. 4486355, RG 85, National Archives, Washington, DC.

Mary Rose: Obituaries, *Los Angeles Times*, June 25, 1999.

Eldene: Author correspondence with Bjorn Paige; Death Record 570-12-1044, Death Master List, US Social Security Administration.

In 1946, Dorothy was stationed through *before he died in 1986*: Author interview with Dan Danner; California Death Index, no. 552106193, State of California Department of Health Services, Center for Health Statistics, Sacramento, CA.

In the 1990s, Dorothy began thinking through *I hear you*: Danner, *What a Way to Spend a War*; Bureau of Medicine and Surgery, "Oral History with Dorothy Still Danner"; author's electronic correspondence with Margie Danner; Arlington Cemetery video supplied by Martin Danner; author interview with Dan Danner.

Bibliography

Arthur, Anthony. *Deliverance at Los Baños*. New York: St. Martin's Press, 1985.

Beaber, John S. *Deliverance! It Has Come! In the Philippines 1942–1945*. University of North Texas Libraries, 2001.

Brines, Russell. *Until They Eat Stones*. New York: J. B. Lippincott, 1944.

Bryant, Alice Franklin. *The Sun Was Darkened*. Boston: Chapman & Grimes, 1947.

Bureau of Medicine and Surgery. "Interview with Bertha Evans St. Pierre, World War II Navy Nurse POW." Oral history with Jan K. Herman, May 20, 1992.

———. "Interview with CDR Margaret Nash, NC, USN World War II Nurse and Pow." Oral history with Andree Marechal-Workman, August 1992.

———. "Interview with Mary Rose Harrington Nelson, Nurse POW, World War II." Oral history with Jan K. Herman, February 17, 1994.

———. "Oral History with Lt. CDR. (Ret.) Dorothy Still Danner." With André Sobocinski, December 3–4, 1991.

———. "Oral History with Pharmacist's Mate Donald Tapscott, USN." With Jan K. Herman, March 25, 1998.

———. "Oral History with RADM (Ret.) Ferdinand Berley, MC, USN." With Jan K. Herman, May 1, 1995.

———. "Recollections of CAPT Ann Bernatitus, NC, USN, (Ret.)." Oral history with Jan K. Herman, January 25, 1994.

Butow, Robert J. C. *Tojo and the Coming of the War.* Princeton, NJ: Princeton University Press, 1961.

Carter, Kit C., and Robert Mueller. *US Army Air Forces in World War II: Combat Chronology, 1941–1945.* Washington, DC: Center for Air Force History, 1991.

Casey, Hugh J. (Maj. Gen.). *Engineers in Theatre Operations: Reports of Operations, United States Army Forces in the Far East, Southwest Pacific Area, Army Forces, Pacific, 1947.* Washington, DC: US Government Printing Office, 1951.

———. *Engineers of the Southwest Pacific, 1941–1945.* Washington, DC: US Government Printing Office, 1947.

Cates, Tressa R. *The Drainpipe Diary.* New York: Vantage Press, 1957.

Chapman, Peter, and Ethel Chapman. *Escape to the Hills.* Lancaster, PA: J. Cattell Press, 1947.

Cogan, Frances B. *Captured: The Japanese Internment of American Civilians in the Philippines, 1941–1945.* Athens: University of Georgia Press, 2000.

Cressman, Robert J. *The Official Chronology of the US Navy in World War II.* Annapolis: Naval Institute Press, 1999.

Danner, Dorothy. *What a Way to Spend a War: Navy Nurse POWs in the Philippines.* Annapolis: Naval Institute Press, 1995.

Edmonds, Walter D. *They Fought with What They Had.* Boston: Little, Brown & Company, 1951.

Flanagan, E. M. (Lt. Gen.) *The Los Baños Raid: The 11th Airborne Jumps at Dawn.* Novato, CA: Presidio Press, 1986.

Giles, Donald T. *Captive of the Rising Sun: The POW Memoirs of Rear Admiral Donald T. Giles*. Edited by Donald T. Giles Jr. Annapolis: Naval Institute Press, 1994.

Ginn, John L. *Sugamo Prison, Tokyo: An Account of the Trial and Sentencing of Japanese War Criminals in 1948, by a U.S. Participant*. Jefferson, NC: MacFarland Publishing, 1992.

Glusman, John A. *Conduct Under Fire: Four American Doctors and Their Fight for Life as Prisoners of the Japanese, 1941–1945*. New York: Viking, 2005.

Gordon, John. *Fighting for MacArthur: The Navy and Marines Corps' Desperate Defense of the Philippines*. Annapolis: Naval Institute Press, 2011.

Hart, Thomas C. *War in the Pacific: The Classified Report of Admiral Thomas C. Hart*. Edited by Charles Culbertson. Boston: Clarion Publishing, 2013.

Hartendorp, A. V. H. *The Japanese Occupation of the Philippines, Vol. II*. Manila: Bookmark, 1967.

———. *The Santo Tomas Story*. New York: McGraw-Hill Book Company, 1964.

Hayes, Thomas. *Bilibid Diary: The Secret Notebooks of Commander Thomas Hayes, POW, the Philippines, 1942–45*. Edited by A. B. Feuer. Hamden, CT: Archon Books, 1987

Henderson, Bruce. *Rescue at Los Baños: The Most Daring Prison Camp Raid of World War II*. New York: William Morrow, 2015.

Hind, Renton R. *Spirits Unbroken: The Story of Three Years in a Civilian Internment Camp Under the Japanese, at Baguio and at Old Bilibid Prison in the Philippines from December 1941–February 1945*. San Francisco: J. Howell, 1946.

Jeffrey, Betty. *White Coolies: A Grim Account of Australian Nurses in Japanese Hands*. London: Richard Hill Printing, 1958.

Johnson, Judith. "Laura Cobb: A Kansas Nurse in a Japanese Prisoner of War Camp." *Navy Medicine* 94, no. 1 (2003).

Kentner, Robert, PhMlc, USN. "A Daily Journal of Events Connected with the Personnel of the US Naval Hospital, Canacao, PI from the Outbreak of War in the Philippine Islands, 12-8-1941 until Liberation of Bilibid Prison, 2-8-1945." Hospital Corps Archives, Bureau of Medicine and Surgery, Bethesda, MD.

La Forte, Robert S., Ronald E. Marcello, and Richard L. Himmel, eds. *With Only the Will to Live: Accounts of Americans in Japanese Prison Camps, 1941–1945.* Wilmington: Scholarly Resources, 1994.

Lapham, Robert, and Bernard Norling. *Lapham's Raiders: Guerillas in the Philippines, 1942–1945.* Lexington: University Press of Kentucky, 1996.

Lawton, Manny. *Some Survived.* Chapel Hill: Algonquin Books, 1984.

Lucas, Celia. *Prisoners of Santo Tomas.* London: Leo Cooper Ltd., 1975.

MacArthur, Douglas. *Reminiscences.* New York: McGraw Hill Book Company, 1964.

Maga, Timothy P. *Judgment at Tokyo: The Japanese War Crimes Trial.* Lexington: University Press of Kentucky, 2001.

Matloff, Maurice, and Edwin M. Snell. *US Army in World War II: Strategic Planning for Coalition Warfare, 1941–1942.* Washington, DC: Office of the Chief of Military History, Department of the Army, 1953.

Monahan, Evelyn M., and Rosemary Neidel-Greenlee. *All This Hell: U.S. Nurses Imprisoned by the Japanese.* Lexington: University Press of Kentucky, 2000.

Morton, Louis. *The War in the Pacific: The Fall of the Philippines.* Washington, DC: Center for Military History, 1953.

Nash, Grace C. *That We Might Live.* Tallahassee, FL: Nash Publications, 1984.

Norman, Elizabeth M. *We Band of Angels: The Untold Story of American Nurses Trapped on Bataan by the Japanese.* New York: Random House, 1999.

Owens, William A. *Eye-Deep in Hell: A Memoir of the Liberation of the Philippines, 1944–5*. Dallas: Southern Methodist University Press, 1989.

Redmond, Juanita. *I Served on Bataan*. Philadelphia: J. B. Lippincott, 1943.

Rubens, Doris. *Bread and Rice*. New York: Thurston Macauley Associates, 1947.

Sams, Margaret. *Forbidden Family: A Wartime Memoir of the Philippines, 1941–1945*. Edited by Lynn Z. Bloom. Madison: University of Wisconsin Press, 1989.

Schaefer, Chris. *Bataan Diary: An American Family in World War II, 1941–1945*. Houston: Riverview Publishing, 2004.

Schwartz, John L. "Experiences in Battle of the Medical Dept. of the Navy," pt. 2, "Pearl Harbor." In *History of the Medical Department of the US Navy*. Washington, DC: US Government Printing Office, 1953.

Sides, Hampton. *Ghost Soldiers: The Epic Account of World War II's Greatest Rescue Mission*. New York: Anchor Books, 2001.

Stevens, Frederic H. *Santo Tomas Internment Camp: 1942–45*. New York: Stratford House, 1946.

Tanaka, Yuki. *Hidden Horrors: Japanese War Crimes in WWII*. Lanham, MD: Rowman & Littlefield, 2017.

Todd, Carrie Edwina. "Nursing Under Fire." *Military Surgeon* 100 (April 1947): 335–341.

Utinsky, Margaret. *Miss U*. San Antonio: The Naylor Company, 1948.

Vaughan, Elizabeth. *The Ordeal of Elizabeth Vaughan: A Wartime Diary of the Philippines*. Athens: University of Georgia Press, 1985.

White, W. L. *They Were Expendable*. New York: Harcourt, Brace and Company, 1942.

Wygle, Peter R. *Surviving a Japanese P.O.W. Camp: Father and Son Endure Internment in Manila During World War II*. Ventura: Pathfinder Publishing Company, 1991.

Yenne, Bill. *The Imperial Japanese Army: The Invincible Years, 1941–42*. New York: Bloomsbury, 2014.

Index

Page numbers in italics indicate illustrations